WORKING OUT IN A CITY THAT WORKS YOU OUT

A perfect guide to fitness

Kobi Noiman

authorHOUSE®

AuthorHouse™ UK Ltd.
500 Avebury Boulevard
Central Milton Keynes, MK9 2BE
www.authorhouse.co.uk
Phone: 08001974150

First published by AuthorHouse 5/21/2009

ISBN: 978-1-4389-4270-4 (sc)

Library of Congress Control Number: 2009902321

Printed in the United States of America
Bloomington, Indiana

This book is printed on acid-free paper.

Contents

Introduction

Welcome to the wonderful world of fitness – a truly remarkable word. Fitness, according to the Webster's dictionary, is defined as the state or condition of being physically fit, esp. as the result of exercise and proper nutrition. To become physically fit you must first become stronger. That is stronger in more ways than one – mind, body and spirit. The majority of the people I have seen over the last 8 years do not have a sense of what training really is. How can they really be doing cardio while watching the television set and/or talking on the cellular phone. Are they for real? How can they really be out of their comfort zone? The minute you step foot into a gym, fitness center, fitness facility or any other type of fitness related room a switch has to ignite – a new person comes to life. That person is fresh, committed, motivated, determined, disciplined, dedicated and invigorated. Their goal has to be within reach and very realistic or tangible; this way it is something they can actually witness, feel and appreciate. They must tune out all interruptions, distractions, negativity and fear. It is the perfect balance between visualization and realization. Visualizing your sole duty in the gym and realizing that you will soon achieve your goals. These two components alone will help aid drastically in your pursuit to that body you always wanted and pictured yourself in.

So now that we got some basics down you need to be comfortable with who you are now. When I say now, I mean at this particular moment while you're reading this book. Since the body is dynamic and always changing you must understand that your goal is not too farfetched. Your body has gone through numerous amounts of changes since childhood, so why not change it one last time. Change it to fit your needs; make it the body you always wanted and desired. For I guarantee you once you change it to your preference you will never change it back. Treat it as such – it is your shrine so do not let up. With this course of action, other factors will immediately come into play. If you change it to your preference you will never change it back. You will begin to gain confidence, pride, strength and a great sense of accomplishment. You are now coming to grips with your overall appearance, attitude and views on the new "YOU."

With all this said and done, allow me to introduce myself. Fitness by Kobi, owned by master trainer kobi Noiman, is a well established and popular training studio in Brooklyn, NY. We offer nothing but the best of trainers, advisors and nutritionists. I consider my studio a fitness consulting group of personal trainers who pride themselves on being leaders in the fitness industry. Fitness by Kobi is a facility built on the principles of dedication, discipline, determination and will. These principles are yours to keep forever and ever. My place is where our reputation lies in the transformation of your body, health and overall manifestation. We are always meeting your needs and exceeding your expectations.

This book will provide you with endless information, training programs, tips and techniques to achieve your perfect body. I will go through many exercise routines, and supply an array of photos showing how to do each exercise with proper form. The biggest mistake you can make in the gym is not doing the exercise properly and listening to others who don't know much about correct form and control. You must first start off as a beginner and gradually climb the latter to become a fitness guru. It is a tall ladder which I am still climbing but my knowledge and experience will help put this book together. With all this said and done I hope you enjoy what I have to offer and begin your quest immediately. There are always excuses and delays so I only ask that you don't give in to them and separate yourselves from those who do. "Fitness is not a luxury, it is a necessity."

I have been around gyms and all sorts of trainers for almost 10 years now. I guess you can call me a gym junkie. I trained with some of the best trainers in the industry and also had the privilege of training with some of the absolute worst. Almost anybody now wants to become a trainer – the profession is real lucrative. I mean where else can you pick your hours, train people who pay you lots of money, workout in between clients and enjoy looking at some of the nicer clients that walk into the gym? It's the ideal job; however not every trainer is the ideal trainer. Trainers are a dime a dozen – all I can say is if you're in the market for a trainer check his/her credentials and qualifications (more about trainers in chapter 1).

So as previously mentioned I am a gym junkie and have had my share of ideas, speculations, theories, and experiments and came across much more literature than you can imagine. Therefore, I felt compelled to write this book and share my knowledge with those who are willing to learn. This book will not be filled with models and bodybuilders posing and demonstrating how to do an exercise, it won't have any fitness jargon and it sure will not be made up with medical terms. Fitness is not a made up thing and it is very realistic and has to be treated like anything else. I am not a big fan of all these books that involve using a dictionary and seeking words and terms that I don't ever hear being used in a gym. I am writing this book with the intent that my readers are just like me when it comes to fitness and do not have the time to constantly seek information from the internet or some other source. I would like this book to serve as a catalyst for many things – a few of these things all come with the beginning of becoming fit (ex. Health, motivation, determination, dedication, power, strength, purification, prioritization, commitment, will, appreciation and many more). There is only one problem with fitness and here it goes: once you embark on the path of becoming fit and healthy it is no longer a once in a while thing. You are now married to this lifestyle forever. No excuses, no lies and no looking back. You owe it to yourself to continue because giving up is much easier than actually going the distance.

Since I have been working out and learning about the fitness industry and the direction it has gone, I decided that a book would be of great justice to many. My credentials are fairly high – Certified Personal Trainer, proud gym owner (Fitness by Kobi), gym designer too many clients, fitness cover model, competed in a number of natural bodybuilding shows, lecturer to children and adults with eating disorders. I figured the next step for me to convey what I have to offer and say would have to come in the form of a book. I am extremely happy that many of my clients sanctioned me to personally publish a book that serves as a guide for overall health. I am grateful that they see my potential and continue to push me and market myself to so many others that have yet to hear about me. This book and what will go into this book will make up a fitness blueprint for the reader. It will be a blueprint in the sense that it will give them the foundation for the process of transformation. I will make this book easy to understand and at the same time interesting. It will be something that every reader, everywhere in the world can relate to. Almost like one of those things that you say to yourself, 'Oh yeah I know what he is talking about!' I can only say that I wish there was a book like this when I first embarked on my beautiful, yet very challenging, path to achieve overall perfection in my body. I began at age nineteen; yes I was a late bloomer, and read books and magazines that contained images of Arnold Schwarzenegger. Arnold is the absolute truth when it comes to fitness; an absolute icon and genius in every sense of fitness. I was blown away at his images and even more appalled at what he offered in terms of being fit and healthy and reaching his ultimate goals. Once turned pro bodybuilding/Mr. Universe/Mr. Olympia/Movie Star/Author/Hollywood mogul, Arnold used many of his principles which he learned from bodybuilding and climbed up a very huge ladder (considering he was 6 feet). He had perseverance, dedication, will, and the absolute desire to achieve indescribable goals. He is no different than you and I. In fact he is just an excellent example of how a human being can obtain whatever he/she desires. Thanks Mr. Schwarzenegger!

Before I start getting into all the specifics and details of weight training, I would just like to leave you off with this:

"Fitness is not a luxury, it's a necessity." It is something that we all can do. Excuses for living a healthy life and incorporating fitness into your life should not be tolerated or spoken of. It is like speaking of your loved one in a negative way or tone. I will only tell you about my experiences and others as a way to maybe motivate you or inspire you. I am in no means a true author of fitness, let alone a fitness mogul or some superstar. I am real, I am like you. The only difference that we share is the love for fitness. Like I said before, and I will mention it periodically in this book that fitness for me constitutes who I am. It is my DNA – it binds me together. It is for me as close to reaching my ultimate high. As the world revolves in an ever changing manner we begin to take things for granted. We become so intertwined in our lives, never really understanding what or who we are. We become so self-absorbed in our daily routines that we watch time just pass us by. Often thoughts and ideas linger, but aren't really satisfied. These ideas never go into action only because we are already planning what the next day has in store for us. So like many of us we just continue to do what it is that we do best. Everyone has their niche – their absolute passion for something. However, there are many who go their whole lives not knowing what they strive for; better yet not even able to experience a burning desire for something or someone. Since we are so self involved in our daily account of events we get side swept and just shove everything to the side.

I guess we all become or became creatures of habit. The question that I have is, are we the ones who set these habits or did we inherit them? Think about this while reading this book and begin to make some changes. After all you already made one change by picking up this book and reading this far. So go ahead and begin to embark on a journey into the wonderful world of fitness.

Chapter I
Basics

Part I - Basics

Weight training has many beneficial components. The overall advantage that weight training has to offer is the improvement on one's quality of life. It helps strengthen bones, boosts energy levels, helps burn fat, gain muscle, and increases confidence levels. It is one of the healthiest activities you can pursue and enjoy. On the other hand it can also be a frightening experience. If you know how to use every single piece of equipment and have a perfect nutritional background then you should be fine! However, that is not the case for many of us out there. With all the different types of machines and equipment, the lingo and rules one can easily get discouraged and lose all hope. Many people I come across are usually frightened, intimidated, concerned, uncertain and usually not so motivated. Therefore, it is important that a book like this be put into use. I want to know that my readers are walking into the gym holding this book and making sure that before they tackle on fitness and weight training they are fully knowledgeable. Its fine to make constant references and go over a few things – everyone needs a little help after all. Ask and you shall receive. Seek and you shall find. You will receive endless amounts of useful information based on experiences, trial and error and expertise. Seek what it is you're looking for and you will find. All it takes is just a commitment. A real sense of pride to begin something that we all take for granted – HEALTH. As previously mentioned, this book will be as easy to read as I can make it. I will go over all the basic jargon, choosing a quality rated trainer and gym, workout routines and many different exercises you can perform for each body part. It will be broken up into sections that all concentrate on weight training. Sections like machines and their functions, anatomy, nutrition, exercises and many useful photos. I will go over equipment that I believe is useful and effective. Remember there are many manufacturers and many different types of machines. Every gym, studio, fitness center is equipped with machines that they think best serve their clients. Upon designing my personal fitness facilities I knew the clients that I would be catering to and so therefore chose my equipment with ease. I knew one place will be strictly for young adults and men who enjoy working out. Hence, I decided to furnish my gym with Life Fitness and Hammer Strength machines as well as a huge amount of Dumbbells, Barbells and cable attachments (all of which I will explain shortly). The same goes for you, the reader, pick your gym carefully and have an idea as to what you want to achieve. If its yoga then make sure it's a nice quiet atmosphere that caters to yoga. If they're bodybuilders make sure the Dumbbell rack goes higher than 70 pounds. Those looking for only cardio make sure that it has every single piece of new cardio machine for you to use. In general, always have a plan and always follow the plan out to its maximum potential.

Many questions relating to weight training often go unanswered. People are always seeking information and unfortunately not all information they receive is 100% accurate. Personal trainers, nutritionists, consultants and others are always there for your assistance but are not always accurate. From my experience many preach to their clients what they believe works either because it worked for them or it worked for others. That is not the case with me – I became a good trainer by being able to differentiate my workouts and my routines with those of my clients. I always tell my clients that what once worked for me does not work for everybody. Everybody is totally different from head to toe and who am I to tell you what I think works best. People can give you advice, tips and even knowledgeable recommendations but in the long run no one knows your body better than you. Always remember that and you shall prevail. This is a common mistake for a beginner and can either steer him/her in the wrong direction or just discourage them. Everyone is quick to offer free advice – they feel like they possess some type of quality that you don't. That is why I published this book – my guidance is highly appreciated and because of it I was able to write this book and run two very successful fitness facilities. I would recommend though keeping your eyes and ears open because along the way you will learn something useful and true from some individual. This actually leads to the second part of this chapter.

Part II – What constitutes a good trainer? What do I look for in a trainer?

This book offers detailed instructions for numerous amounts of exercises with enough knowledge to give you confidence to workout on your own. Still, many will seek trainers as a means to motivate them, educate them, or just go over some basics that they don't seem to grasp. So choosing a trainer who is suitable for you is not an easy task. Should you just pick the strongest trainer in the gym? Or better yet maybe the trainer that looks good and poses in some magazines? A trainer must have some credentials for you to decipher amongst a few other trainers. They have to stand out like any candidate applying for a job. How does their resume look? Are they highly experienced? Are they certified from an accredited university or organization? Can they really motivate you or are they just in it for the money and status? These are just a few thoughts that should enter your mind before you make a decision.

A fitness trainer or personal trainer has become famous for firming up all sorts of people, from movie stars, models, professional athletes and so many others. With the current trend that fitness is heading in a personal trainer is not that bad of a job. However, since just about everybody can become a trainer this makes the process of choosing one difficult. A good trainer has to be educated (in his/her respected course of study), able to perfect your techniques, keep you focused and motivated – never letting your goal disappear, quick on their feet (this refers to what I love – improvisation), show that they are different in many aspects and can even be able to carry a normal conversation with you. I don't mean someone to talk to you about nonsense the entire session but someone who can carry a normal conversation and entail other items than fitness. Versatility is a great quality and you should look for that. Do not be so quick to pick the first trainer that walks over to you or corrects your form, there is so much more than that. Trainers in gyms are like sharks in the water – just waiting for fresh meat to arrive. Since you are paying for your trainer experiences make it worth wild. Every dollar spent should be put into good use.

Many commercial gyms and even private health clubs and studios require that their trainers have at least one certification. This is a good standard that may set one trainer apart from the other and may guide you in picking the right trainer for you. Many private/freelance trainers are earning certifications with many organizations as a way to stay ahead of the increase in competition. The more certifications the better, education has no boundaries. If you see a trainer with more than one certification, chances are he/she is a great trainer because they enjoy learning and keeping up with current trends/ideas/etc... Some trainers are just working in this industry to either pay for rent in between their acting careers, make a bit of extra cash and the most famous one I always hear is "you never know who might bump into in the gym." Like trainers, certifications are easy to come by and many on-line companies are offering them for either a small fee or some type of course on the internet. I did none of those and received three certifications the old fashioned way – attending courses, workshops and going to take an actual exam. Below you will find a list of reputable certifying organizations: (you can also do a search on google to find more)

- International Sports Sciences Association (ISSA)

- American College of Sports Medicine (ACSM)

- National Academy of Sports Medicine (NASM)

- American Council on Exercise (ACE)

- National Federation of Personal Trainers (NFPT)

There are a few others, but the ones mentioned above are all accredited and highly recognized. Just so you know, hire an experienced trainer – remember your paying for them so do your homework and research. Try to hire a trainer with a decent personality, I mean after all your going to be with them for an hour so at least enjoy the experience. Be sure to always get personal attention: your trainer should thoroughly evaluate your goals, health, desires, injuries and medical concerns before starting any program. Your goal has to be their main objective and together you guys can reach it quicker. From my experience I always make my client number one. Not only are they my main concern in the gym but I try to extend to the outside as well. An occasional phone call, text message, instant message or email is highly appreciated and the client relates to that. You begin to develop a friendship. A true sense of what you need to help your client succeed. I am direct and straightforward with all my clients and till this day they are number one in my book. After all it is because of them that my studios flourish and this book is published. In addition if there is something you don't know always seek an answer. I am never afraid to tell my clients that I don't know an answer but I always tell them that I will find out. So with that said and done you can begin your process of choosing a trainer immediately. Choose wisely, choose smart, choose logically and get going with your transformation.

Just like there are rules for choosing a trainer there are also some rules for acting during training sessions. Show up on time, all the time. Trainers are also professional people with bills and busy schedules just like you, so show them some courtesy. It will only benefit you to arrive on time so that the full hour is used accordingly. If you're going to be late please notify them in advance and if you're going to cancel give them at least a 24 hours notice. This way they can plan their schedule and/or even fill in your spot. I always let the first one or two sessions slide and did not charge them but not all gyms do. Be responsible and take actions into your own hands. Come to the gym with a good attitude – try to filter out all the negative things. When you're in the gym the only thing on your mind should be gym related. No one cares about your boss, girlfriend, boyfriend, wife, or whatever else you can think of. Give your trainer a 100% attention and in return he will do the same. In addition, if you're not the swift one and memorize everything then do take some notes. Buy a journal and write in it – after all you can always relate back to it. Listen to what your trainer has to say and don't ever be hesitant to speak up. Trainers are not mind readers and will just keep on talking assuming you absorb everything. The more you interact and ask, the more educated you will become.

Chapter 2
Tune in to Your Nearest CABLE Attachments

Every gym or fitness center has many pieces of attachments either somewhere on the floor or hanging off some type of rack. For many, this may look like a pile of metal and crap, but actually very useful. These attachments or steel and rubber looking things are known as cable attachments. They are all used for a cable machine or any pulley machine and can be easily put on and taken off. If you're afraid to go near these attachments start getting used to them and enjoy the unlimited variety of exercises. It will spice up your workouts and even let you have some fun and get creative. Below you find a rundown of some cable attachments and I will notify the popular ones:

Long Bar

These bars come in various lengths and are usually used for back exercises. They can come as long as 6 feet. The longer the bar, the harder the motion becomes. Most of the bars are made up steel and/or metal, but since majority of people I know are concerned with their hand appearance they also come with either rubber grips at the ends or even the whole bar is made out of a rubber substance. The same things go for dumbbells – some are made from steel and others are made from rubber, neoprene and other raw materials.

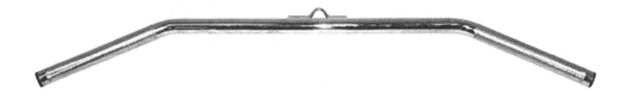

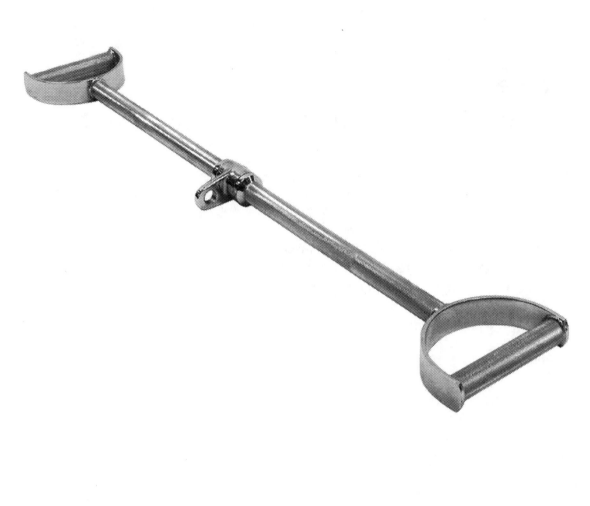

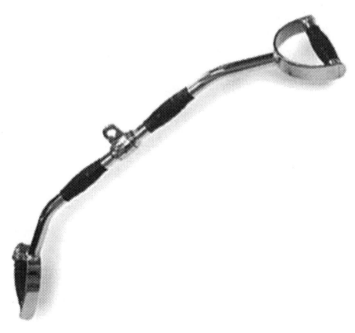

Close-grip bar

These bars are made for a smaller and tighter grip. They are commonly used for back exercises as well. They are great for really developing the muscles by your armpits and your upper back. It is considered a compound exercise/movement and targets the biceps as well.

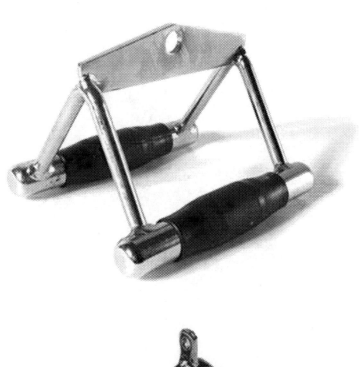

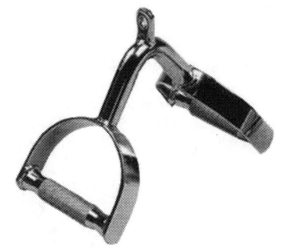

Curved Bar (also known as an e-z bar, a V-shaped bar or a U-shaped bar)

These bars are primarily used for both bicep and triceps exercises. The reason this bar is called an e-z bar is because it is much easier on your wrists and many people I come across have weak wrists and forearms. They are highly effective and in my opinion the most popular used bars. Once again based on preferences they can come with rubber grips at the end so that way it won't give you any calices.

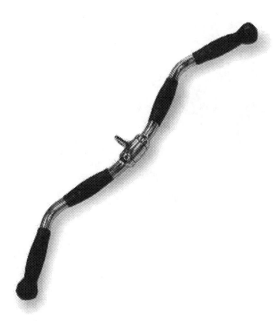

Straight bar - these bars also come in a few sizes – short, medium and long

These bars are also commonly used for bicep and triceps exercises. Great for biceps curls, reverse curls, triceps pressdown and a few others. In addition, these bars can also serve as great exercises for back and shoulders (seated cable row, front raises and a few others)

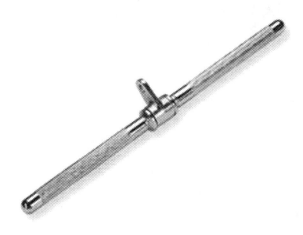

Horseshoe handle or better known as single grip handle

This piece of attachment is a bit different than the others. This is a single handle and you are able to work each bodypart individually. It's used for numerous chest, back, shoulders and arm exercises. I consider this attachment a great piece because it allows the individual to perform certain exercises a bit more strict and controlled. You are working each side individually and you cannot cheat or get help from the dominant hand. Most exercises that require a bar are a bit easier because if you're struggling on one side of the body, the dominant side will take more of the workload. This is the case with so many people that are either right handed or left handed. The dominant arm gets the bulk of the exercise and weight. Both are examples of this handle – one is steel and the other foam padded with a steel grip.

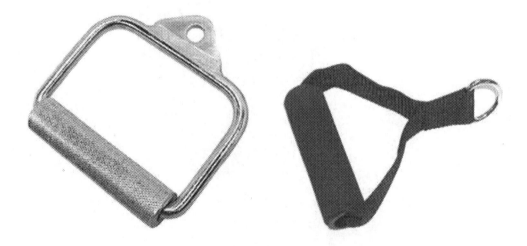

Rope

The rope – commonly used attachment for the triceps. However, it has so many other functions that most are unaware of. For example you can do Hammer curls for biceps with this attachment, front raises for shoulders, and even some abdominal routines. Every gym you walk into will have a few of these ropes at different cable stations, so don't be afraid to grab this rope and experiment a bit.

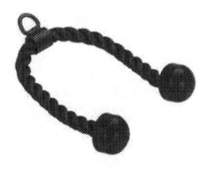

Ankle collar

This is not highly used but is still found in many gyms. It usually comes in either a leather strap, Velcro strap or any type of ankle bracelet that clips onto the cable station to perform exercises such as leg lifts, leg curls and other inner and outer thigh exercises. As a trainer I use this often with my clients but as mentioned before it is not a popular contraption.

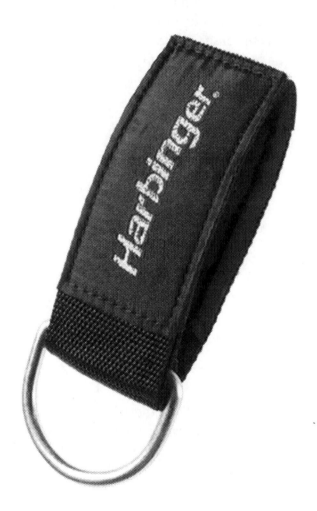

*** Do not think for a minute that these are the only attachments you can find in a gym. There are so many other attachments on the market but for me to cover all of them will only be boring and long. I covered the basic attachments that are highly used and extremely popular.

So now that we tuned in and went over all the useful CABLE attachments, I think it's safe to say that we can now begin working out. So in the next few chapters you will find numerous exercises specified by bodypart.

Part I – key words that will open the door to your workout experience

In the following list, we will define some fundamental words of the weight training lingo.

Exercise – this word refers to a particular movement or a particular range of motion. For example, Dumbbell curls and Squats are both considered exercises.

Repetition – this term refers to a single performance of an exercise. Most people shorten this word and use it as short for **rep.** For example, performing a certain exercise from the start to the finish is known as a completed repetition.

Set – a set is a number of consecutive repetitions that you complete without rest. Once again, it's the number of times you perform the exercise from start to finish. Most exercises are usually made up of 4 sets and each set contains approximately 12 to 15 repetitions.

Program or regiment – this is a broad term that usually lists every aspect of your daily gym routines. It can be written in a journal and contains information such as the number of exercises, sets and repetitions which were performed. These programs can be highly effective in helping you go over your routines. It keeps you organized and you can always refer back to it to see where it is you stand now. Personal trainers usually carry around a program sheet as a means to monitor their client's progress.

Chapter 3
CHEST AROUND – Working Your Chest

Chest is one of those muscles that people incorporate with brute strength. If I had a dollar for every person that asked me how much can I bench press, I would be a millionaire. Chest is one of those muscles that can either grow or stay stagnant. It can take a major pounding but in many instances it is highly hard to achieve a great chest. When it comes to chest exercises you must find exercises that specifically target your body type. Everyone wants to bench press crazy amounts of weight and make ridiculous noises while lifting the weight. Remember, form and control are the key components to increasing overall strength and eventually help you with the most famous chest exercise – the flat bench press.................. How egoistic. Amazing how some people will do almost anything to lift heavy. That includes arching their backs, using too much shoulder and triceps and not getting a full repetition. I guess the more they lift and grunt and scream the more girls will look their way.

The technical name for your chest is Pectorals – which is split into the pectoralis major and the pectoralis minor. You will never step foot into a gym and hear these two words referred to. Rather the short slang name is Pecs. As aforementioned chest, along with the help of shoulders and triceps, is responsible for most of the pushing and pressing motions. Since your chest muscles are among the largest in your upper body, I suggest that you use a variety of exercises to target every area. You can easily change the feel of many chest exercises by either adjusting an angle on a bench, using proper form, utilizing the chest muscle to its potential and even just changing up routines frequently. You want to always get a good pump in the chest and changing your workout routine is vital. So your next question or thought should be which chest exercises should I be doing and how many exercises do I do for this bodypart? Many trainers believe in totally different things, including exercises, sets and repetitions. This is fine because I mentioned that every trainer is different and some more versatile than others. You must first determine what it is you're looking to achieve so that both you and your trainer know their exact role.

For those trying to put on weight and become massive your ideal rep range should be between 6 to 10 and for those trying to either get defined, a bit muscular, toned or just staying in shape, your ideal rep range should be high – usually 12 to 15. On the contrary, if it's just some weight loses you are striving for then I recommend doing every exercise with a high number of repetitions – usually 20, 25 or even 50.

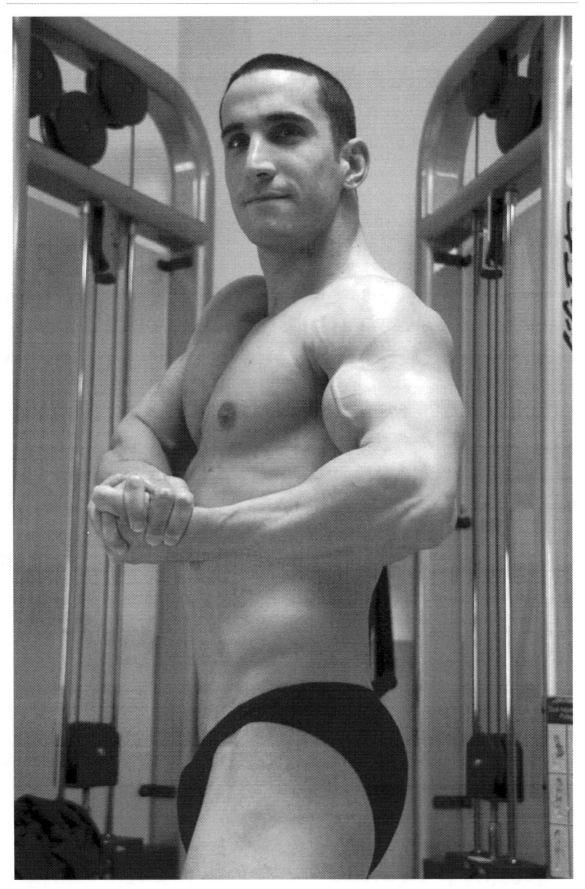

Part I – Exercises

Upper Chest

Incline presses with a barbell, smith machine or dumbbells – all three ways are great for developing mass and strength of the upper chest and front deltoids. Make sure to keep good form on this compound movement and lower the bar until it grazes your chest. When using a smith machine make sure that the bench is positioned accurately and equal in distance from both sides of the machine. In other words, it is extremely important to find the right groove. The same applies for dumbbells – lift each dumbbell simultaneously straight up with palms facing forward and then lower them back to starting position. The lower you go with the dumbbells, the greater the contraction and squeeze you will feel on the upper pecs.

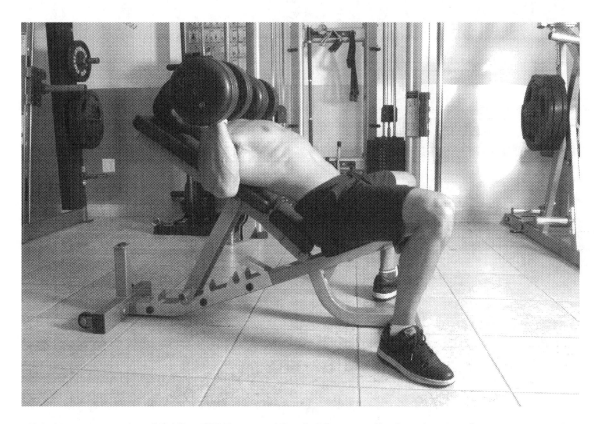

This is an example of Incline DB Presses. See how controlled and strict the movement is.

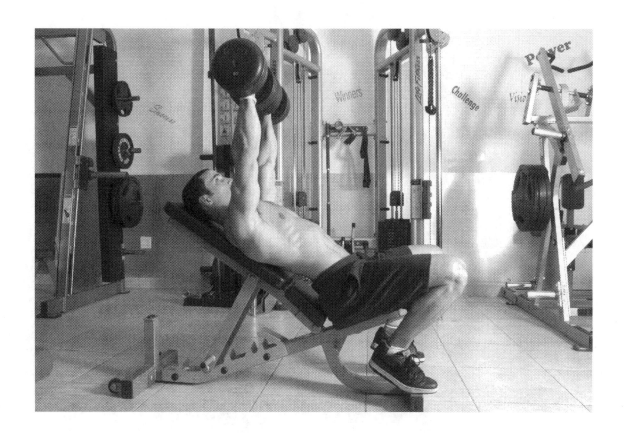

Incline DB Fly's – these fly's are done like any other normal fly's, except for the incline position on the bench. While performing this exercise be sure to hold the dumbbells straight overhead with your palms facing each other. Lower the dumbbells in a sweeping arc keeping the palms facing each other with your elbows slightly bent. I like to tell my clients to pretend that they are hugging their loved ones to ensure strict and correct form. Lower the weights until you feel that your pectorals are fully stretched and come back up through the same wide sweeping arc.

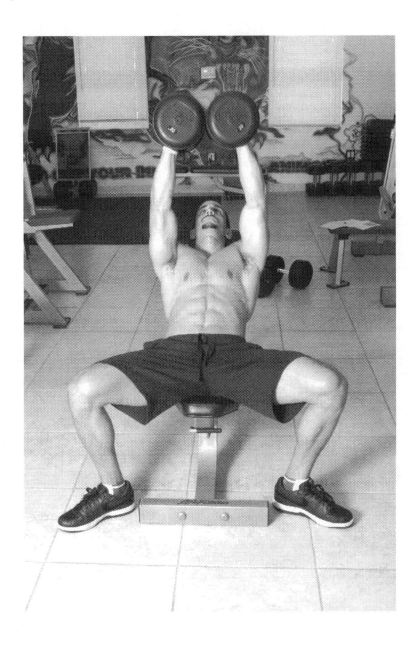

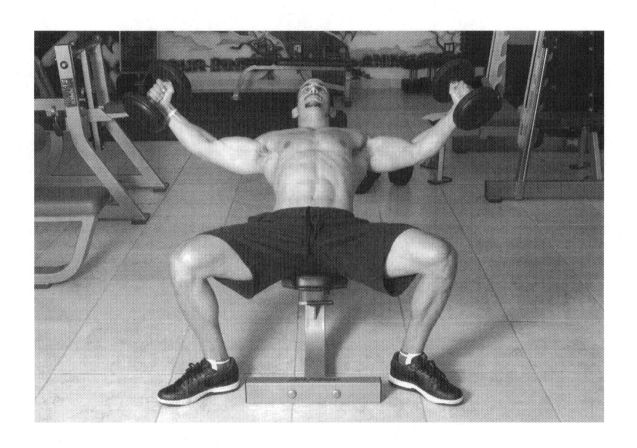

Hammer Strength (Machine) Incline – most gyms have a full line of Hammer Strength Machines that cater to upper, lower and middle chest. They are fairly easy to use and only require you to keep your back on the padded bench and perform the exercise. They are plate loaded so don't be lazy to load and unload weight.

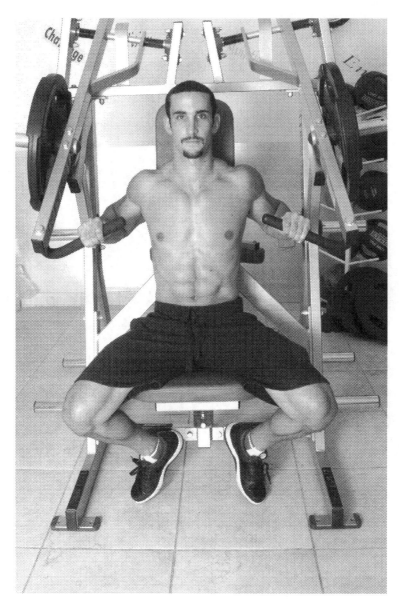

Notice how my neck and back are tightly pressed against the pad. This allows for absolutely no cheating and forces your pectorals to work harder.

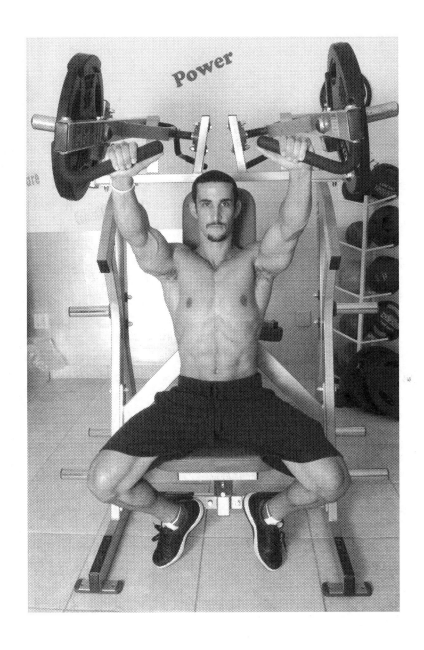

Middle Chest

Flat presses with a barbell, smith machine or dumbbells – once again all three ways are great exercises for developing mass, strength and size of the middle chest. Dumbbells allow for a better range of motion and stability. Barbell is the ultimate power movement and allows for heavy weight while the smith machine is also great for power and strength only with the exception of working on an assisted bar. This bar is attached to the machine and acts as a safety device for all of your movements. You can place heavy weight on the smith machine and go up or down as far as you possibly can before hooking the bar onto the latches. Both the smith machine and barbell are fundamental compound exercises that promote growth, strength, power and muscle density.

-   Barbell – lie on a flat bench with feet either on the floor or on the bench. Take a shoulder-width grip and place it on the bar. Begin to lift the bar off the rack and hold it at arm's length above you and then lower the bar slowly and controlled until it reaches your chest. You want the bar to easily hit your chest or at least be an inch away from your chest and in no means do you allow the bar to bounce off your chest as a form of momentum. Absolutely positively no cheating.

-   Dumbbells – lie on a flat bench with feet either on the floor or bent on the bench. Place a dumbbell in each hand and begin to lift the weights straight up overhead as your laying down flat. Once up in the air and making sure that your palms are facing forward, lower the weights toward the outside part of your chest concentrating on keeping them under control. Lower the weight till you reach a 90 degree angle with your elbows or you can even lower them as far as you can so that way you can feel a complete stretch in the pectoral muscle. Once lowered, begin to press the dumbbells back up to its starting position. Dumbbells are extremely challenging and require much control, balance and stability.

-   Smith Machine – similar to the barbell in all ways except for the fact that the machine can act as your spotter or your training partner. Like I said before, this machine allows you to go heavy while keeping a certain sense of consistency in the motions. Use it wisely and effectively to ensure results.

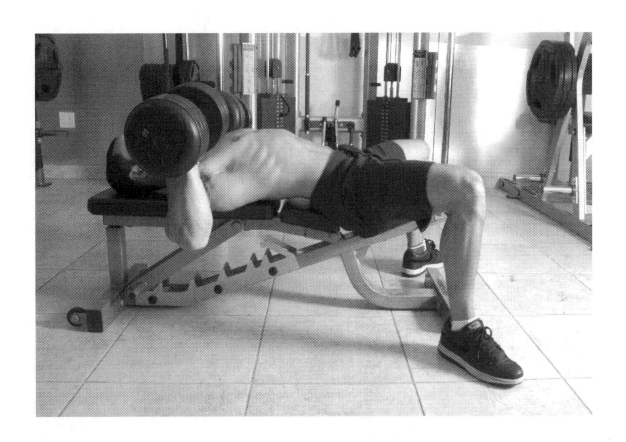

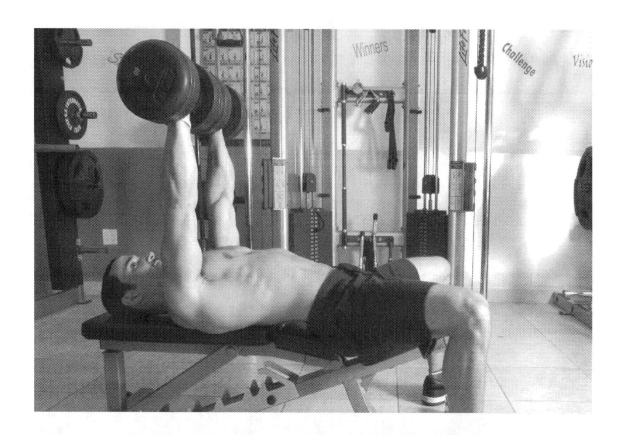

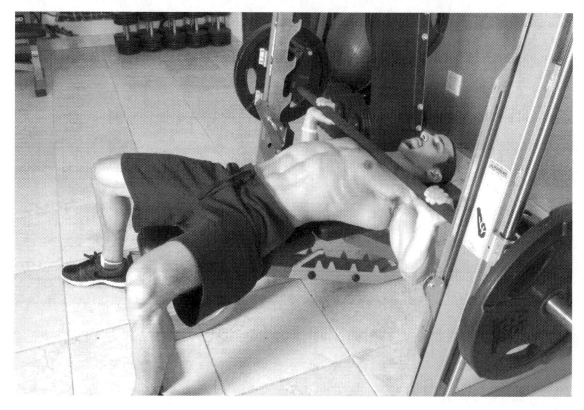

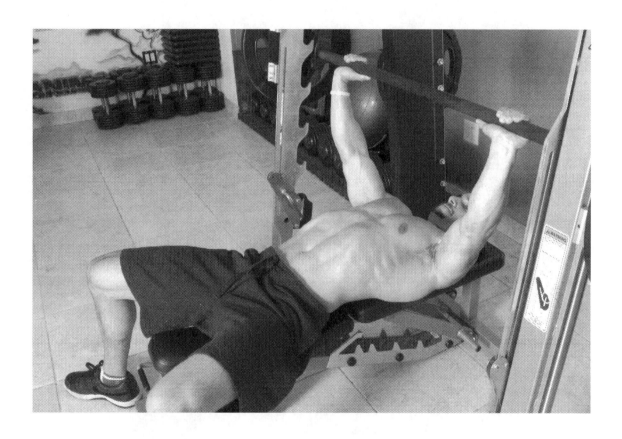

Flat DB Fly's – these fly's are done in the same way that incline DB fly's are done. Lie on a flat bench while holding a pair of dumbbells with your palms facing each other. Slowly begin to lower the weights out and down as far as you can (almost like giving your loved one a hug). The palms should remain facing each other throughout the movement. Obviously the further out you lower the weights the greater the stretch of the pectorals will be. Be wise and make sure your elbows are slightly bent throughout the entire exercise. This will reduce the stress being placed on the elbows.

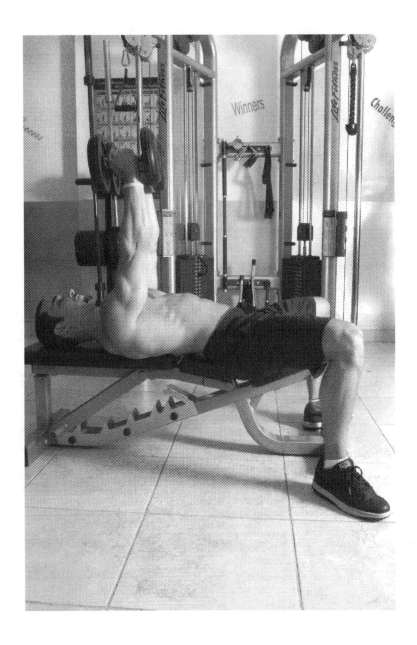

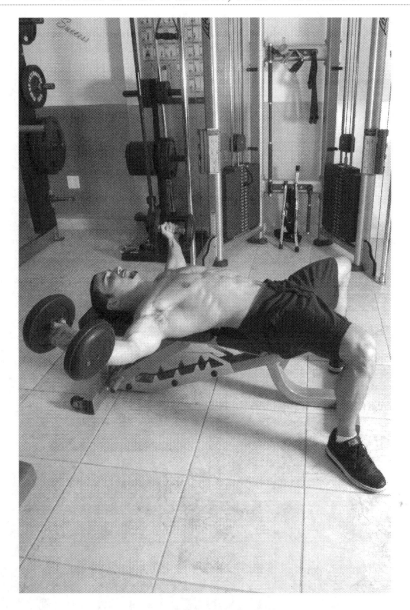

Chest press machine (vertical) – this particular machine is not a power exercise and is mostly used for beginners, those coming back from an injury and rehabilitating or those who don't know much about working out, till now. Sit in the seat of the machine and grip the handles. Begin to straighten your arms while pushing the handles forward and repeat the same motion throughout. To make things more challenging just change your grip on the handles of the machine (close grip, wider grip, underhand grip, etc...).

Lower Chest

Decline presses with a barbell, smith machine or dumbbells - for the last time, all three exercises are great for overall lower chest results. It just becomes a matter of preference and ability. Variety is always crucial for maximum potential and is the spice of life.

This is an example of decline presses with dumbbells – make
sure you control the weight and use strict form.

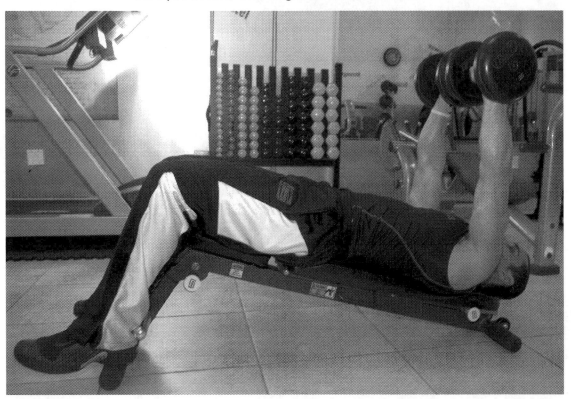

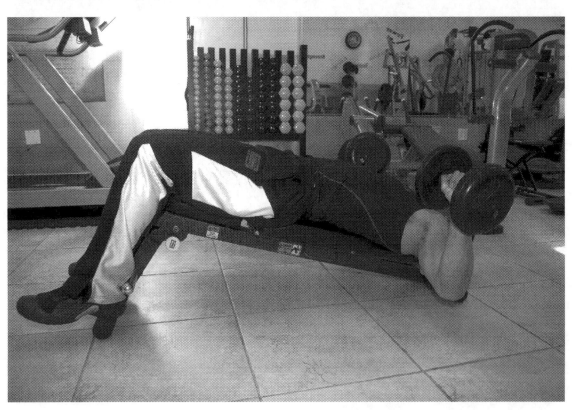

Decline Fly's using dumbbells – this exercise is done just like any other type of fly with the exception of bench positioning. Decline Fly's are great for that lower chest development needed by almost everyone.

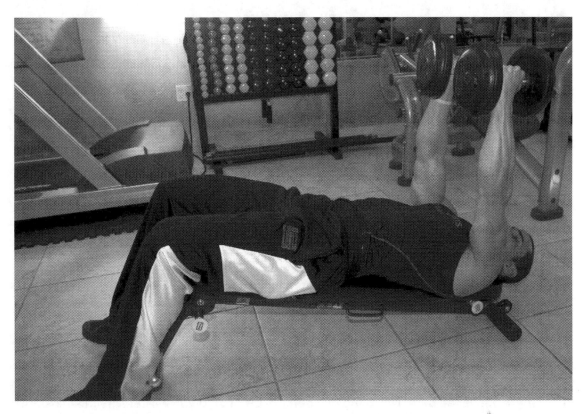

Make sure that you begin this motion with your palms facing each other.

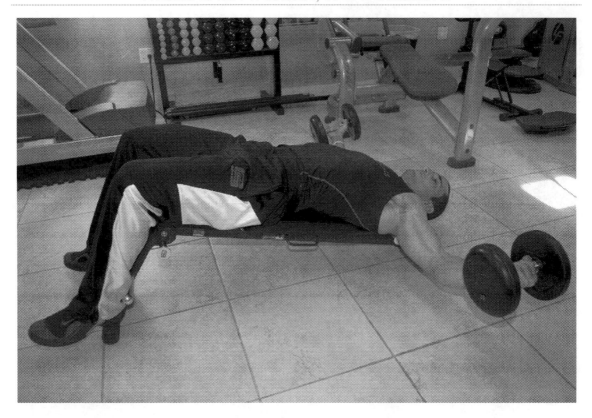

Dips (on a parallel bar dip station) – Dips are great for both the triceps and chest muscles and are similar to many of the decline exercises I have mentioned. The only difference with dips is that you are training with your own body weight. Approach the bars and hold yourself at arm's length above the bars. This is the beginning position and you will feel it almost instantly in your triceps and chest. Begin to lower yourself as far down as you can. Once at the bottom of the movement, start to press back up to the starting position. Make sure that at all times you are tensing and squeezing the pectorals. This exercise can be performed in two ways: facing the machine and facing away from the machine. The further forward you lean, the more chest you involve.

Cable Fly's – this exercise can be done on an adjustable bench and you can easily change the position to better accommodate your needs. In this case we will go over flat bench cable fly's or crossovers. Lie on a flat bench between two floor-level pulleys. If the cable station is an adjustable unit then just lower the pulleys down to the floor. Take a handle attachment in each hand and bring your hands together at arm's length above you. Your palms should be facing each other at the top of this motion. It is exactly the same sweeping arc motion as dumbbells fly's.

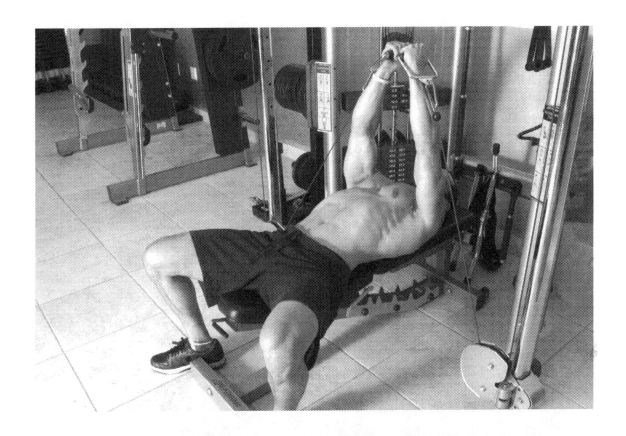

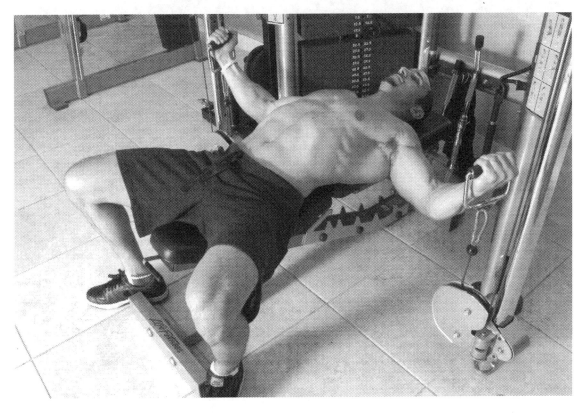

Inner Chest (known as the gap between each pec)

Pec-Dec Fly's or Machine Fly's (both are the same just have different names) – definitely not the best exercise for building mass, but excellent for getting definition and striations. Most gyms are equipped with a variety of these machines. They come in all different colors, different padding and different forms of resistance. I like to consider this exercise as a vertical fly. Always make sure to get the fullest possible range of motion while totally stretching the pectorals to the maximum. This machine is self-explanatory and almost each one has a labeled diagram on the side to better assist you.

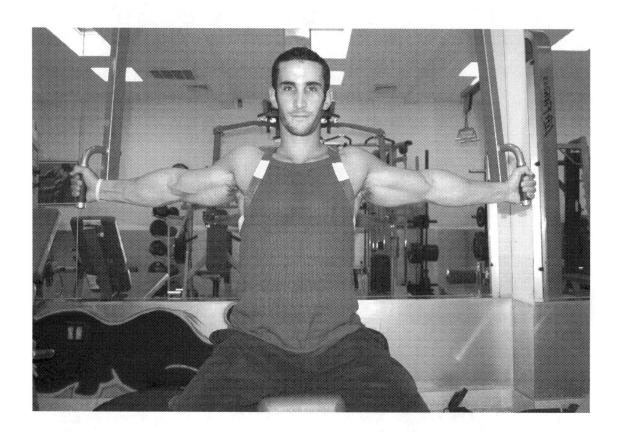

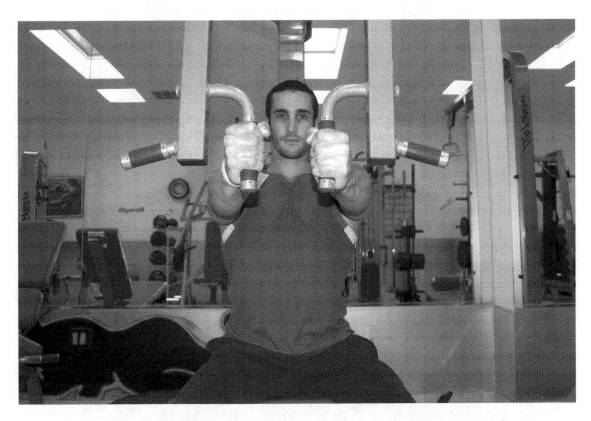

Notice how the middle chest is contracted while doing this exercise – always make sure to use proper form and squeeze the muscle to its full potential.

Cable Crossovers (with a slight contraction at the end) – you want to actually squeeze the muscle after every repetition making sure that the middle and lower chest are being emphasized. This motion is done from a standing position. Take hold of the handles attached to the cable station overhead, step slightly forward with one foot in front of the other for leverage and extend your arms straight out (still maintain a slight bend in the elbows) to either side. Once you're positioned well bend forward slightly from the waist and bring your hands forward and around in a big hugging motion while contracting your pectorals. At the end of the motion your palms should be facing each other and continue to repeat.

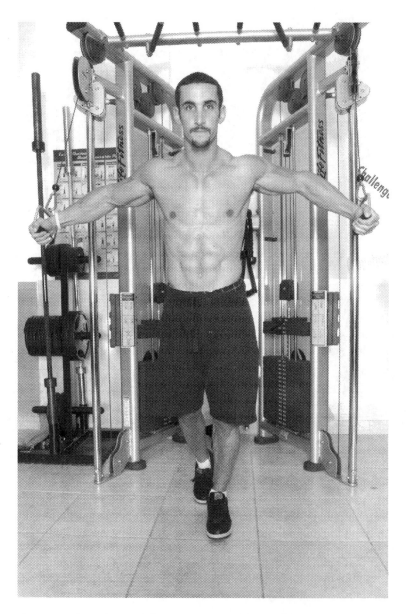

Be sure that the weight is manageable so that way you can
fully stretch out the inner pectoral muscles

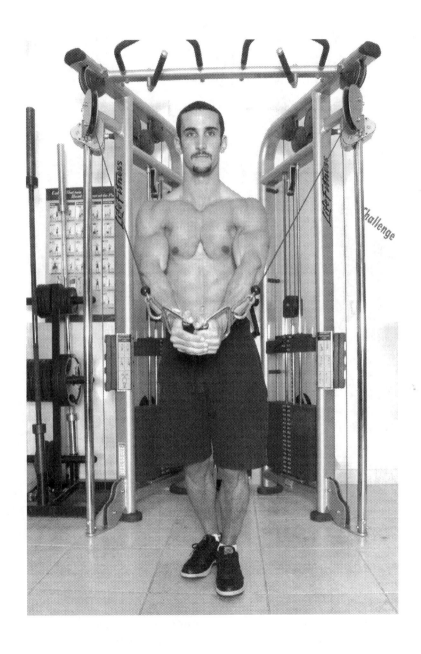

Close Grip Flat Barbell Presses – usually effective for the triceps but also hits the inner chest phenomenally. This exercise is performed like a normal flat bench press with the exception of your hand positioning. Your hands should be about 6 to 8 inches apart to ensure proper contractions for both the inner chest and the triceps. In addition, this exercise could be done with an e-z bar or any other fixated weight barbell.

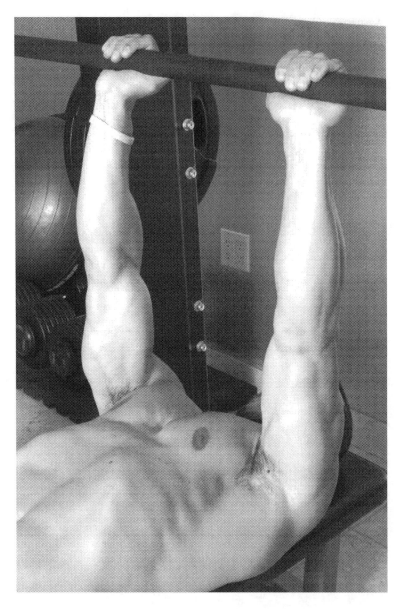

The hand positioning is vital for overall chest and triceps development. If too much stress is placed on the wrists then maybe use wrist pads or decrease the weight.

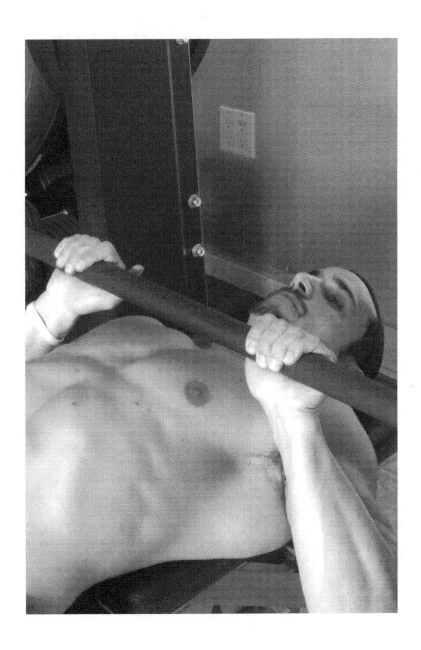

Close Grip or Diamond push up – also very effective for developing triceps, this style of push up is good for developing the inner chest and is a common exercise. However, do not think for a moment that this push up is easy, in fact it is a more advanced form of push up's.

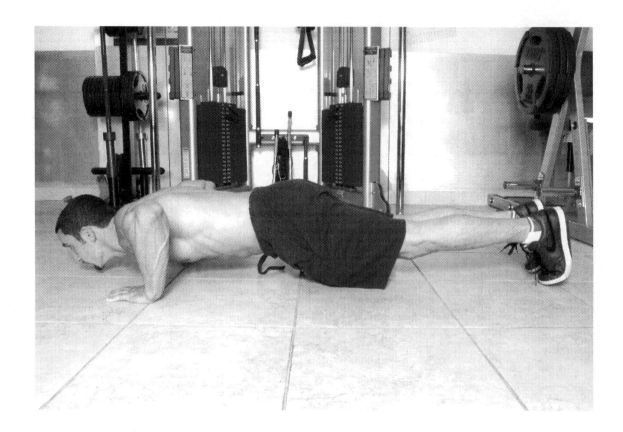

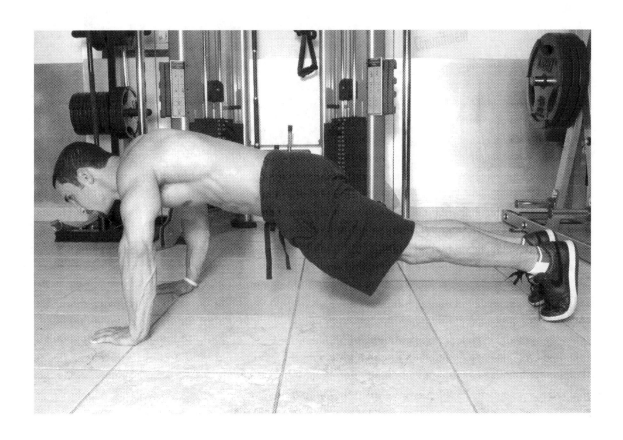

Dumbbell Pullovers – the purpose of this exercise is to expand the rib cage and develop the overall pectoral muscles. Using a flat bench take a dumbbell with both hands and hold it straight up over your chest. The easiest way to explain it is what I call cupping the dumbbell, which means that both palms are pressing or holding the underside of the dumbbell. Keeping your arms straight you begin to lower the dumbbell down in an arc behind your head while feeling your rib cage and chest totally stretch. Once you have lowered the dumbbell as far as you can, raise it back to the starting position through the same arc. Not really a common exercise but I appreciate its development and the way it develops my rib cage and serratus muscle.

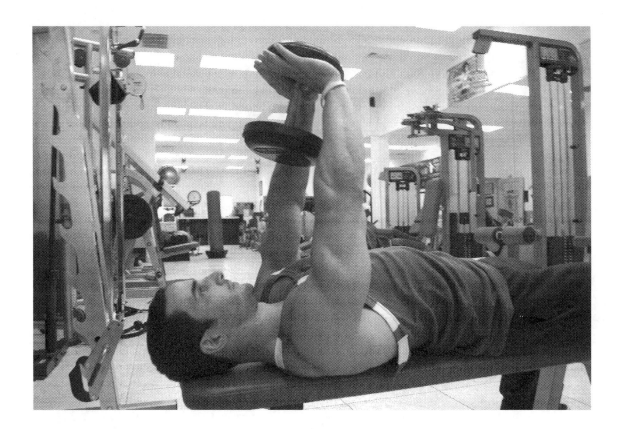

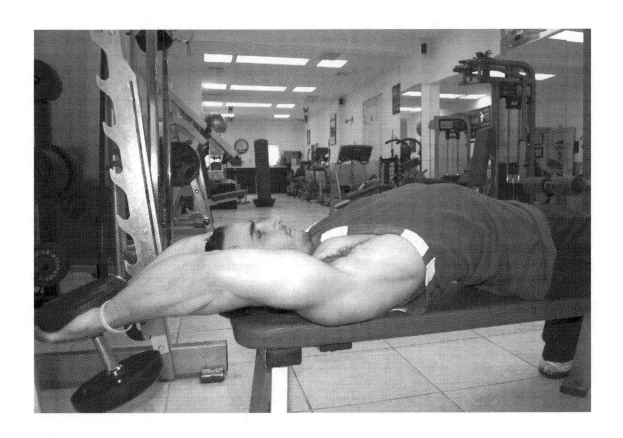

Chapter 4
BACK UP – Working Your Back

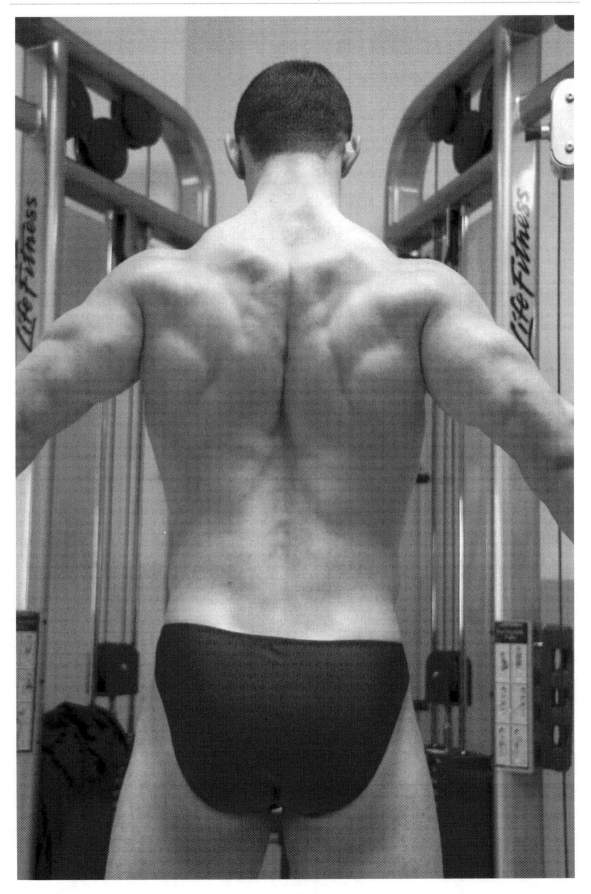

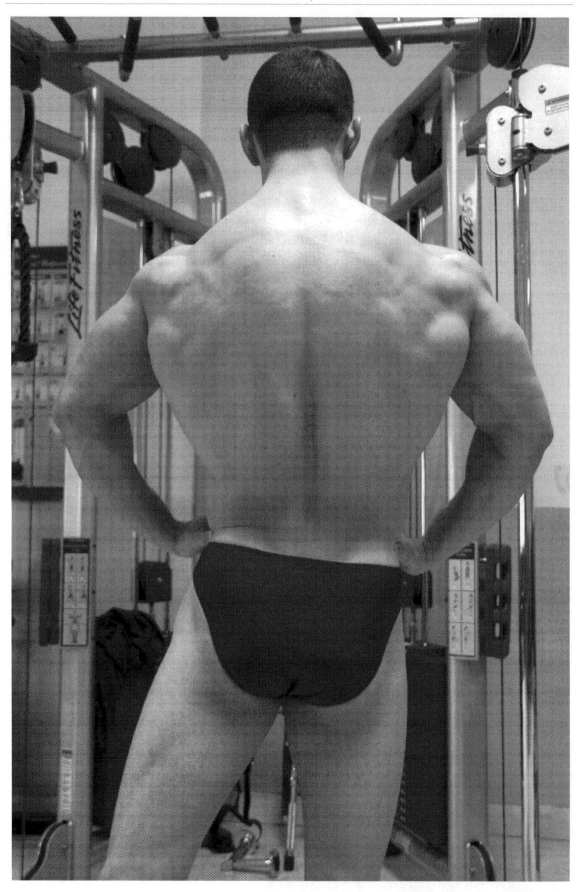

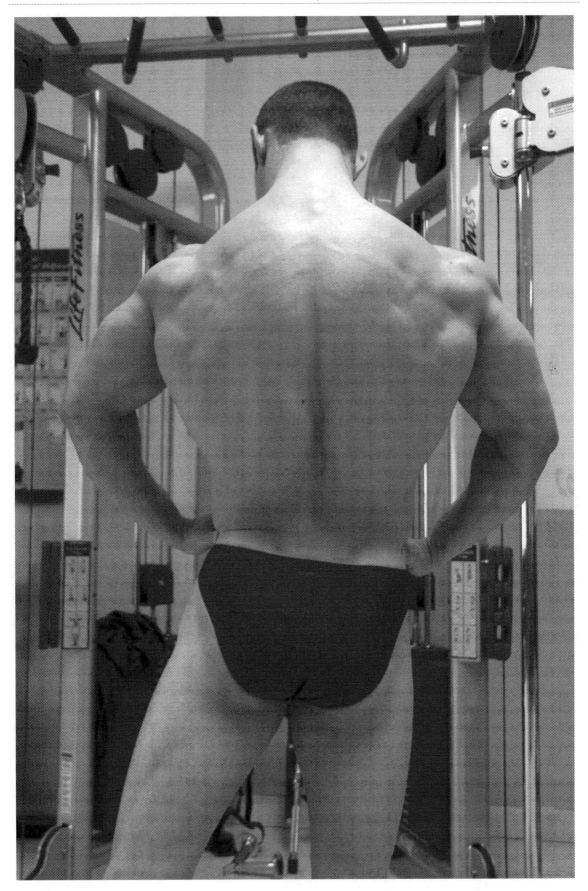

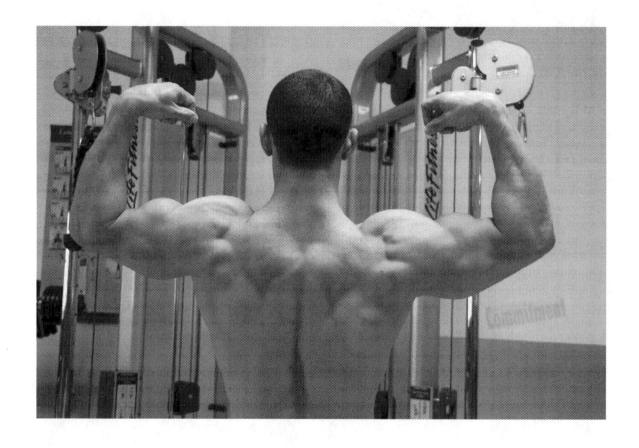

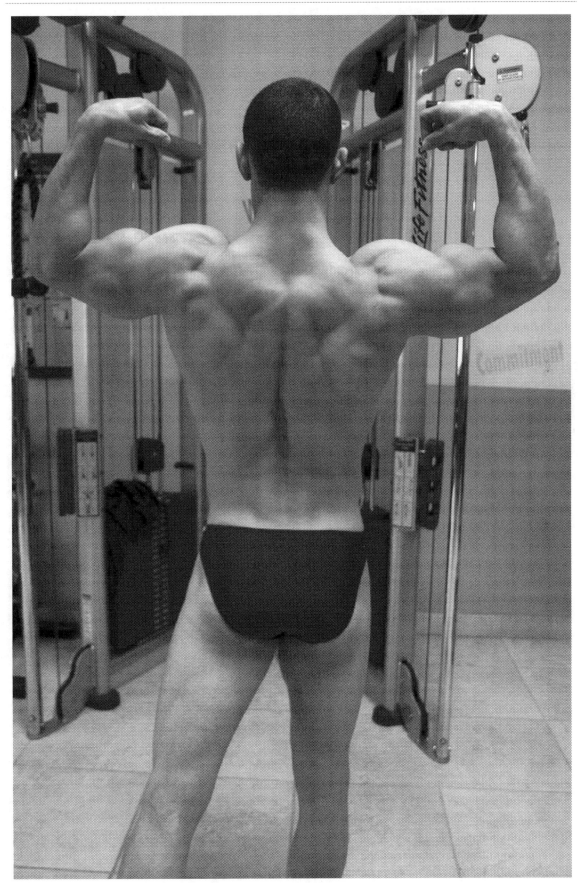

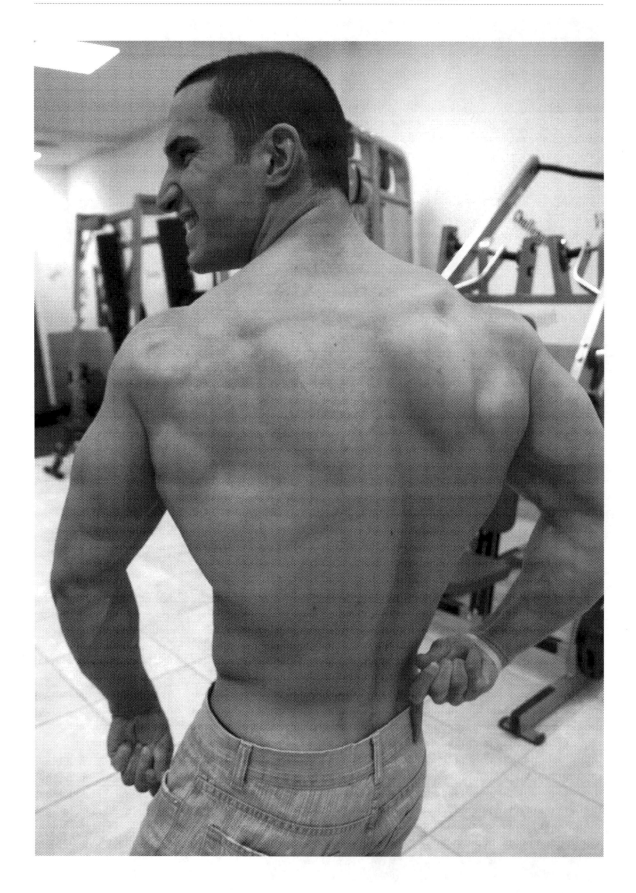

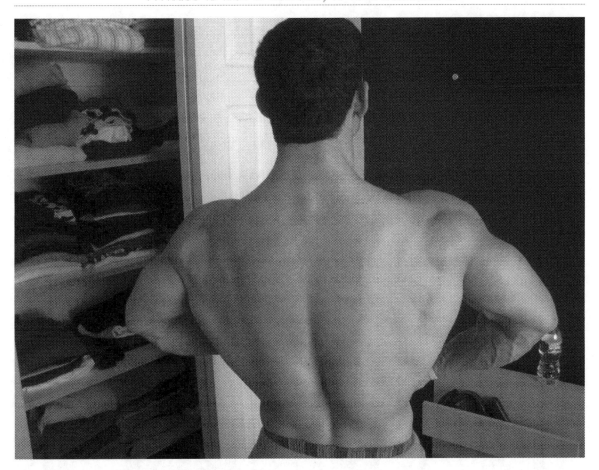

You know those things you use all of your life to pull your arms toward your body, well those are known as your lats. The **Latissimus Dorsi, or lats for short,** is the largest muscle in your upper body. They run from the armpit down to the center of your lower back. Your lower back is made up of **spinal erectors –** these are the several muscles in the lower back that guard the many channels and nerves which help keep the back erect. The back muscles for me were always very interesting and absolutely a joy to work out. The burning sensation you get from doing certain exercises are indescribable and need to be experienced. A great back or a well defined back are very important to overall strength and consistency. Throughout my numerous bodybuilding competitions I can't begin to tell you how important the back muscles are – most of the poses require using and displaying your back such as spreading your lats wide open so that you can nearly fly away. I will go over many exercises for the upper back (lat pull downs), middle back (T-bar rows) and finally lower back (hyperextensions).

Upper Back and Lat's

Wide-Grip Chin-Up's (Pull-Up's) – this exercise can be performed in two ways: either to the front or to the back. Begin by a chin up/pull up station with an overhand wide grip. Hang from the bar stretching the whole area of the back and pull yourself up. A complete motion is one where your chin clears the bar or you are able to touch the top of your chest to the bar. Once you reach the top of the movement you then lower yourself back to the starting or hanging position.

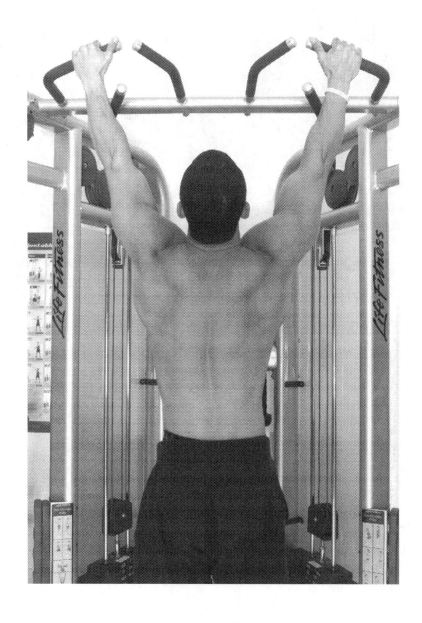

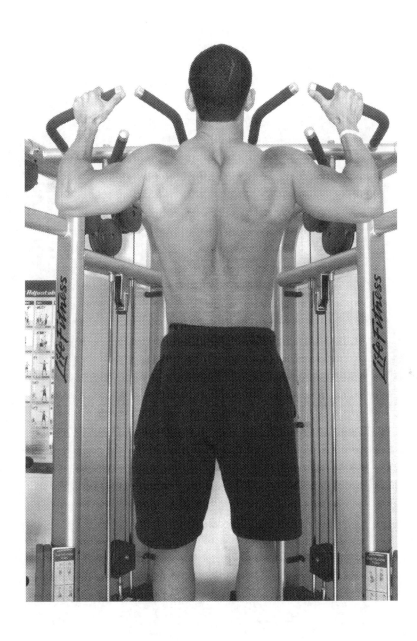

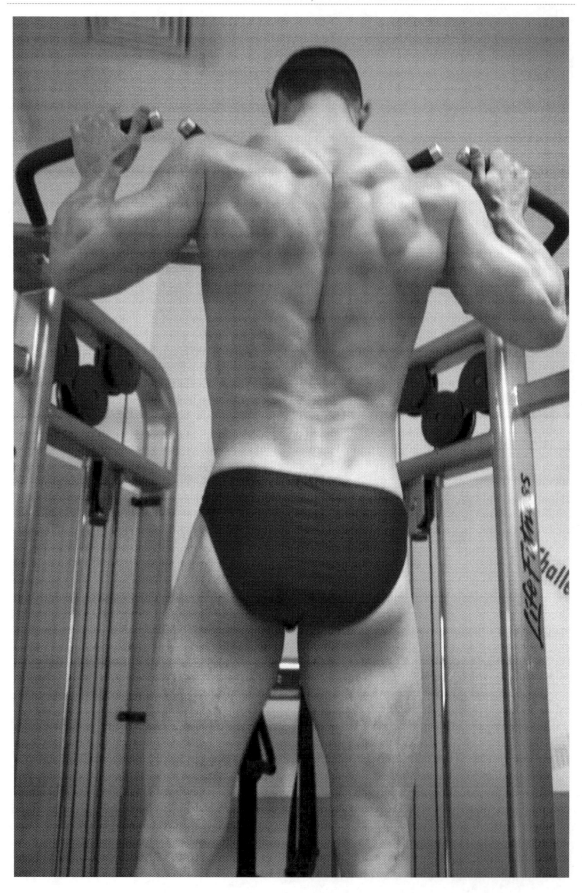

Close-Grip Chin-Up's – this exercise is performed the same way as the wide-grip with the exception of your hand position. This involves your hands being close together with one hand on either side of the bar (v-bar, triangle bar or any other close-grip bar)

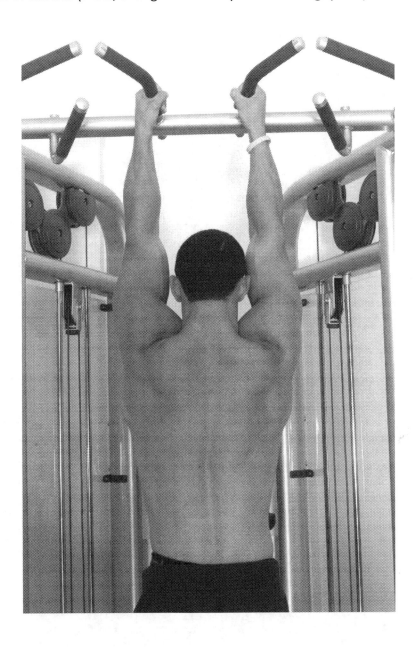

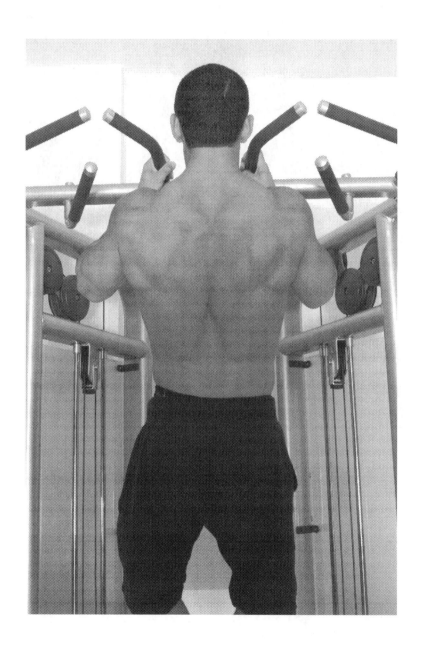

Lat Pulldowns – any wide attachment is suitable. You begin this exercise by taking a wide grip on the bar and taking a seat with your knees hooked under the supported pads. Pull the bar down in a smooth, controlled motion until it touches the top of your chest. Once the bar is lowered and your shoulder blades are contracting start extending the arms back to their starting position. For variety you can do lat pulldowns behind the neck instead of to the front.

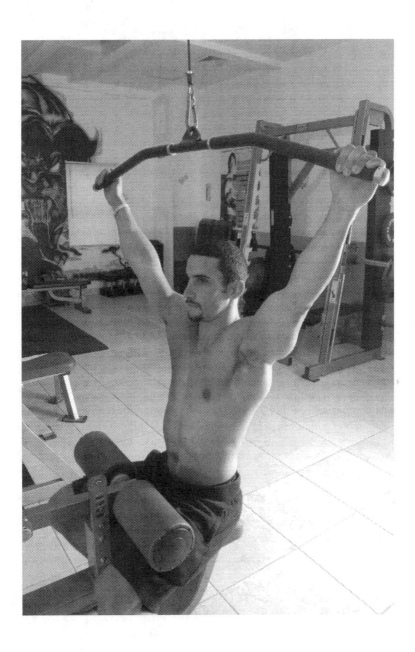

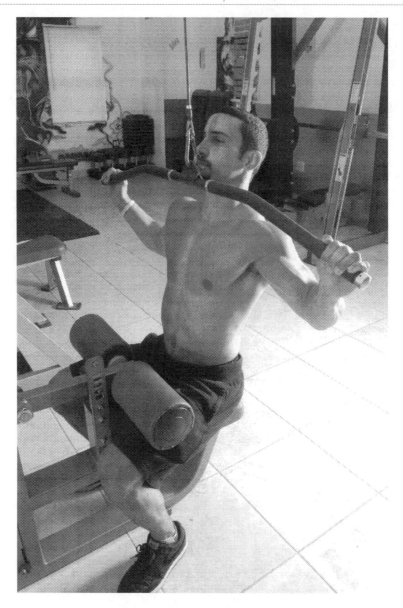

Bent-Over Barbell Rows – this is a powerful exercise which is great for thickening and widening the upper back. Stand with your feet a few inches apart and grasp the bar with a wide overhand grip. Bend your knees slightly and bend forward until your upper body is almost parallel to the floor. Make sure you keep your head up to alleviate pain from the neck and lower back and allow the bar to hang at arm's length below you. Once you feel a great stretch in the lat's and middle back, lift the bar upward until it touches your upper abdominals and then lower it again under strict control back to the starting position. I can't stress how important it is to make the back work and not make it a biceps exercise. Thus, make sure to never bring the bar up to the chest area so that you reduce the role of the arms completely. I personally always started this exercise with a real light weight to totally warm-up and avoid injury.

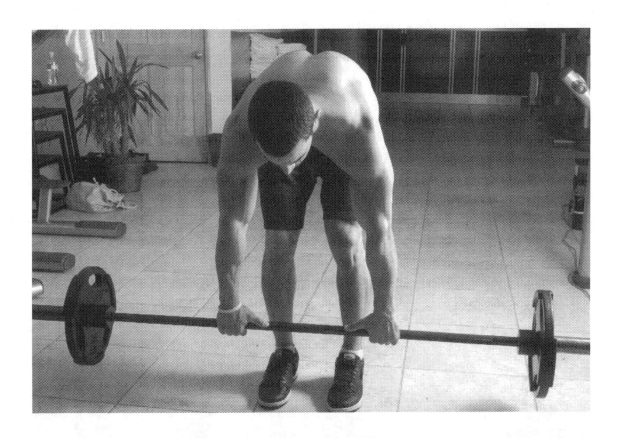

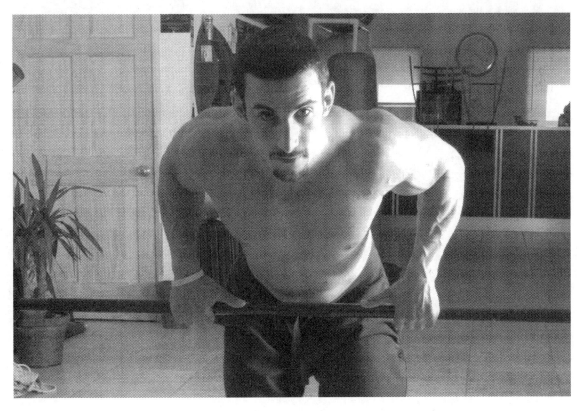

Bent-Over Barbell Rows (under-hand grip) – highly effective form of rows that bodybuilder and hall of famer Dorian Yates loved to do. Same steps and technique as the barbell overhand grip. You should be a professional by this point, so don't pretend like you don't know how to perform this movement.

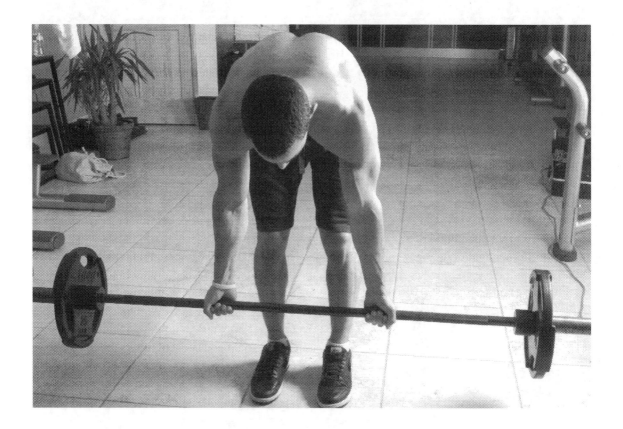

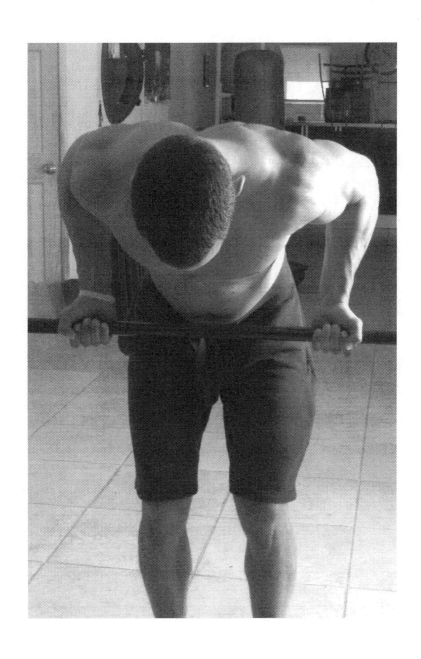

One-Arm DB Rows (two ways) – you can either place your foot on a bench or do what I call "free-standing" rows. Take a dumbbell in one hand, bend forward from the waist until your upper body is nearly parallel to the floor. Place the other hand (the free hand) on the bench as a form of support. In other words, opposite knee of the arm you're working on the bench. You begin with the weight hanging down at arm's full length and lift the weight up to your side. Make sure that your back is steady and that you are concentrating on doing the work with the back rather than the bicep. Finish your repetitions with one arm and then repeat with the other arm.

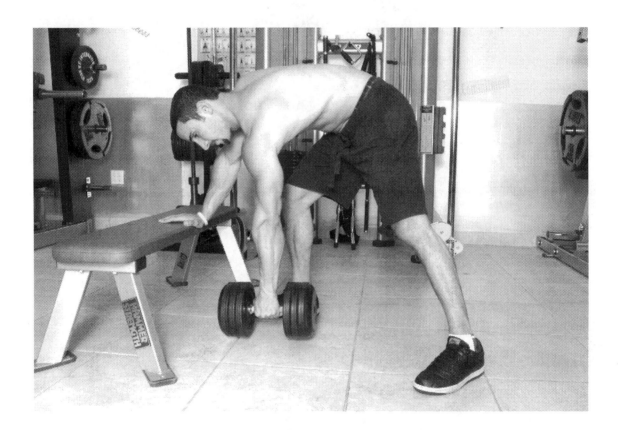

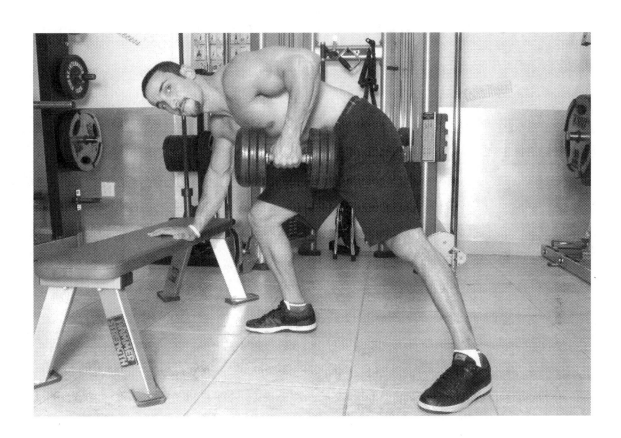

Middle Back

Close-grip Chin-Up's

Seated cable Rows (any close-grip attachment) – the smaller the attachment like straight bar or a v-bar the more you will be hitting your middle back including your rhomboids. The wider the attachment the more lats and the outside part of the back is what you will be targeting. It is good to change attachments regularly so that your body doesn't get used to one particular movement.

Machine Rows (try to hold it in a close-grip distance) – these machines are found in many gyms and are easy to operate. They are self explanatory and always have a diagram posted on the side of the machine to better assist you. The most common machine that I notice in gyms are the Hammer Strength Machines. These are excellent for overall back development.

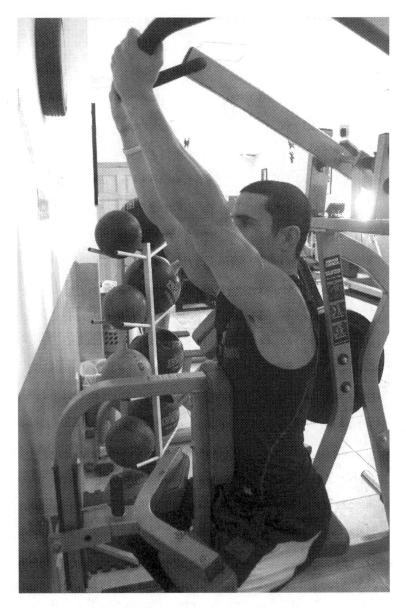

Make sure that your arms are fully extended at the top to ensure maximum contraction and an overall stretch of the lat muscles.

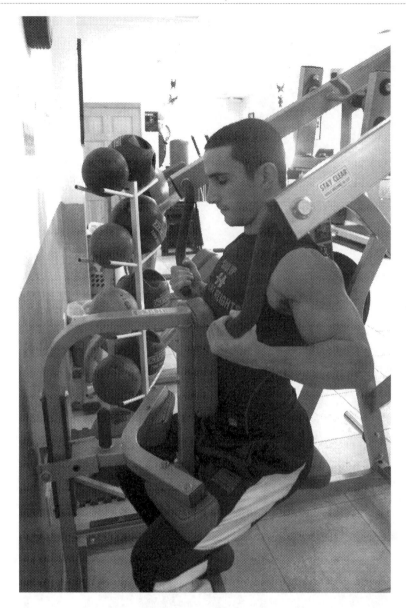

Also be sure to keep your chest against the pad for strict and controlled movements.

T-bar Rows – great exercise for thickening the middle of the back. Most gyms have a fairly modern T-bar row machine and might look a bit intimidating. Start by standing on the contraption with your feet close together and knees slightly bent (make sure you get as comfortable as you want). Bend down and grab the handles of the T-Bar machine/unit with either an overhand grip, a close grip, or an underhand grip. Now that you have a grasp on the bar begin to straighten your legs slightly and lift the bar until your body is at about 45-60 degree angle. Without any changes in your body and angle, lift the weight up until it touches your chest and then lower it again to arm's length. Make sure that the weights never touch the floor so that you have direct and constant tension on the back. Remember, this is a middle and upper back exercise so you are not supposed to do much lifting with the lower back, legs or biceps.

Lower Back (a strong lower back is extremely important in helping you perform strenuous exercise listed above)

Dead-lifts - one of the absolute best exercises for lower back, upper back, the hamstrings, the butt and the trapezius muscles. Dead-lifts are a power movement that requires you understanding perfect technique so that way you don't get injured. This is done by you placing a barbell on the floor in front of you with already loaded plates. Bend your knees, lean forward and grasp the barbell in a shoulder-width grip with one arm in an underhand grip and the other in an overhand grip. Make sure to keep your back straight so that way you don't strain. Once your grip is established and you're back straight, begin to straighten up your body until you get into a standing upright position. Once upright and at attention, lower the weight, bend your knees, lean forward (from the waist while keeping your back straight) and allow the weight to touch the floor before beginning your next repetition. The majority of this exercise involves you driving the weight up with your legs and lower back.

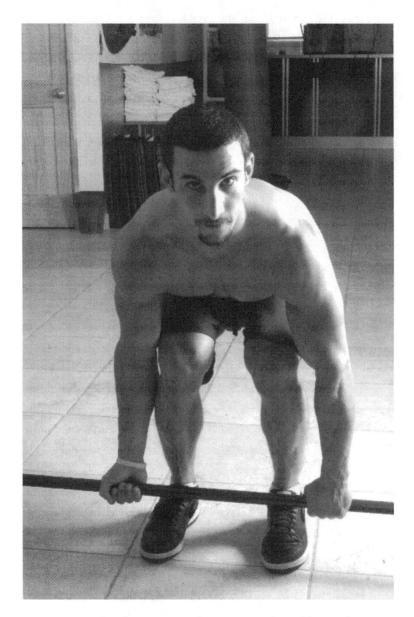

Start (Make sure you have a comfortable grip)

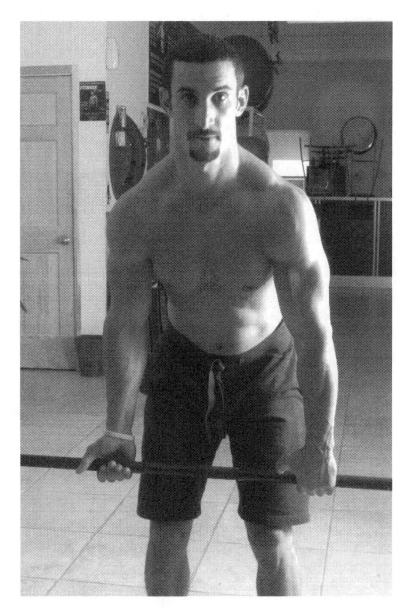

Middle of the motion

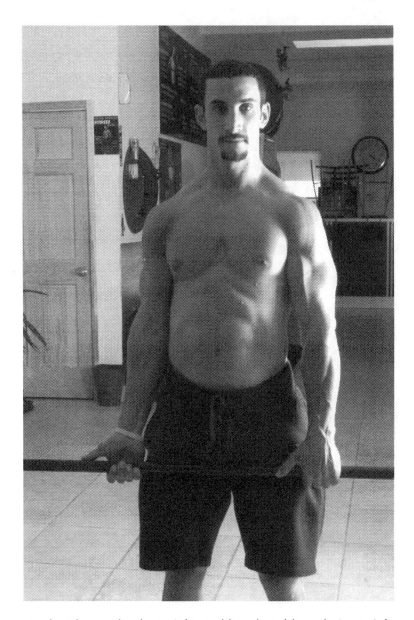

End with your back straight and head up (then do it again)

Hyperextensions – great exercise to develop the spinal erectors of the lower back. You begin this exercise by starting off facedown with your thighs on the pads and heels hooked under the rear padding. You can place your hands across your chest or behind your head and begin to bend forward going down as far as you can until you feel the lower back muscles getting stretched and tight. I like to explain to my clients that on this exercise all they are doing is tucking their body in while going down. From the down position, or tuck position, begin to come back up so that your torso is just above parallel and not any higher.

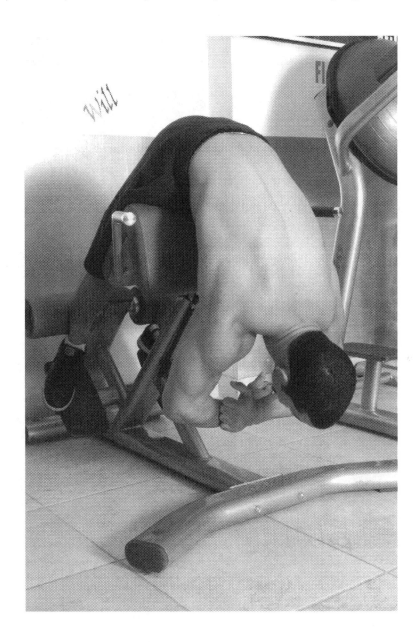

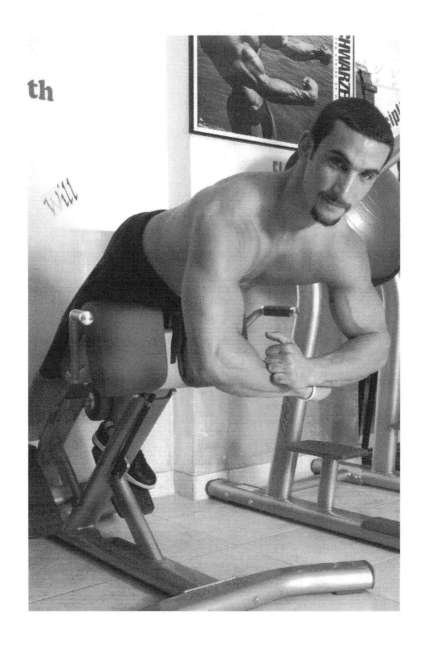

Good-Mornings' – this exercise is almost never used and not common at all. I enjoy this exercise and it gives me a great stretch in my lower back. Find a weight (barbell) that is manageable and place it over your head and on the back of your shoulders. Stand with your feet a few inches apart (bit less than shoulder width apart) and make sure that your legs are locked and your back is straight. From this point on begin to bend forward from the waist with your head up until your torso is parallel to the floor. Go ahead and hold that for a second or two and come back up to the starting position.

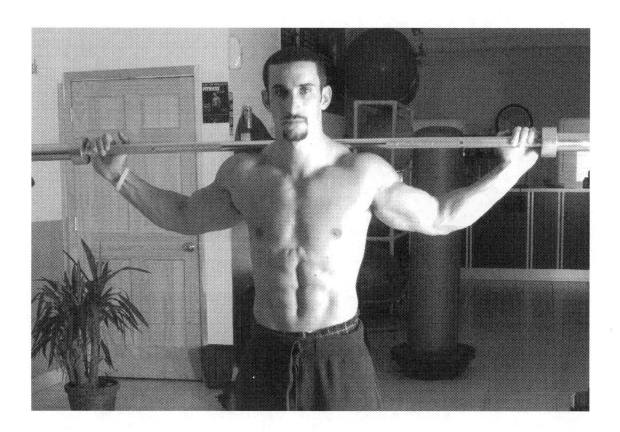

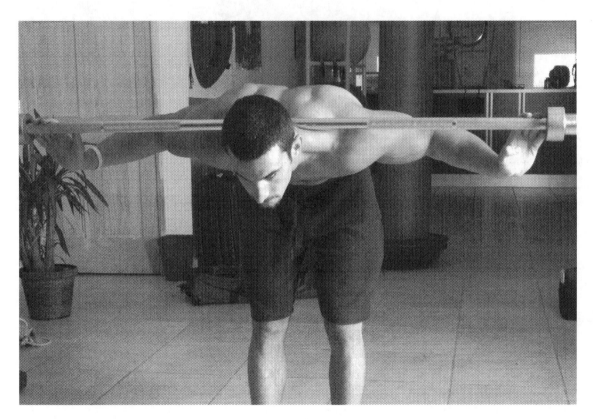

Make sure to keep your head up throughout the movement
to avoid placing any stress on the lower back

Chapter 5
SHOULDERS AND BOULDERS
(Working Your Shoulders)

We all heard this saying before: "if you get broad or big shoulders then your waist will look a whole lot smaller." I heard this saying so often during my younger years as a bodybuilder and always believed that it was true. The Shoulders consist of your deltoids and the trapezius muscle. The deltoids consist of three thick large boulders or what some call heads: The front deltoid, side deltoids (lateral delts) and rear deltoids or posterior deltoids. The trapezius muscles are the most recognized muscles in the upper back region which tie together the neck, deltoids and lat muscles. The trapezius is an important muscle for many poses and holds a lot of weight in most pre-judging instances. Since the shoulder area has many different heads and muscles it is important to make sure that your routines and exercises are done with precision and always changing. I always lean more towards free weights and dumbbells rather than machines when working out shoulders. I think that the free weights give you such a better range of motion and control than machines. I mean don't get me wrong, I love machines and think they are just as great. However, in the case of shoulders, machines should only be used if you are either coming back from an injury or rehabilitating, lazy to load and unload the bar, or just intimidated by the vast amounts of free weight machines. I assure you that these machines are extremely beneficial to your workout routines once you know how to properly use them. Hence, this book will guide you in more ways than one.

So as previously mentioned, the shoulder area is comprised of three unique and very achievable deltoids. Below, you will find the many different exercises you can perform for each deltoid:

Front Deltoids

Military Barbell Presses (standing or sitting) – take a shoulder-width grip of the barbell and begin to lift it off the rack and straight up. This movement also involves your triceps. Once the weight is straight up you can begin to lower it all while keeping it under control.

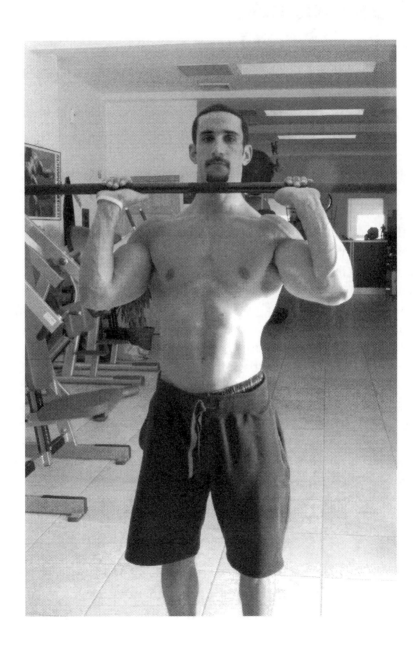

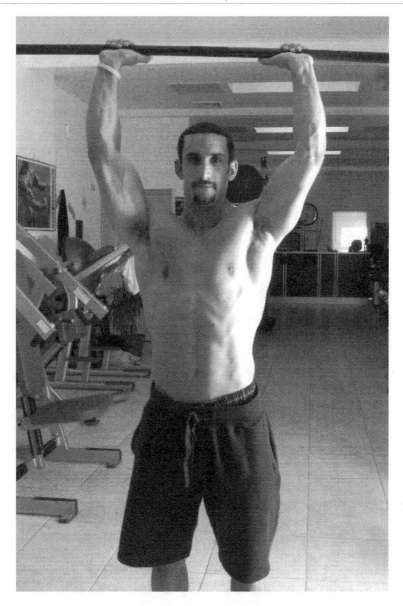

Notice on this exercise I demonstrate standing military presses with a barbell. My hand positioning is pretty close but I do recommend you to hold it at shoulder-width distance. I was preparing for a big show that time and wanted to concentrate on my triceps so I did most exercises in a close grip position.

Smith Machine Presses (seated) or Push Presses (standing) – both are great exercise and both emphasize all three delts beautifully. The smith machine is a great way to go heavy and feel a bit more secured as opposed to the standing barbell push presses. In addition, you can let the weight come down much lower on the smith machine which in essence places a greater stretch in your front delts.

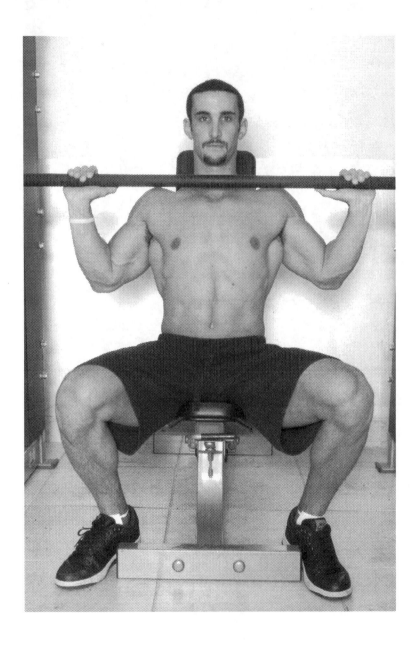

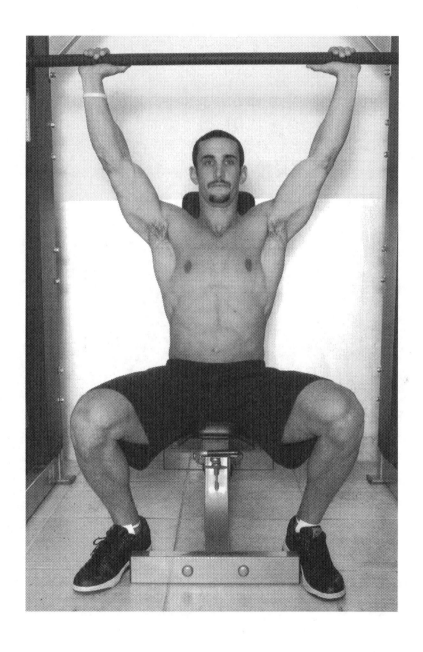

Dumbbell Presses – definitely a great way to stress all three deltoid heads. Hold a dumbbell in each hand at shoulder height with your elbows out to the side and your palms facing forward. This is known as the starting position. Begin to lift the dumbbells straight up until they touch at the top of the motion and then lower them to about a 90 degree angle. This is known as the finish position. The major difference with dumbbells is the greater range of motion you can get.

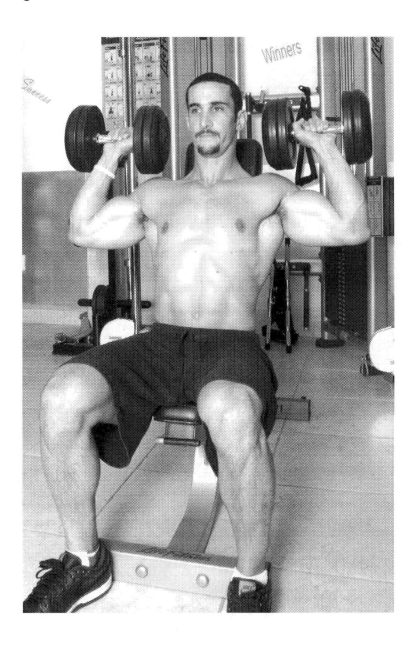

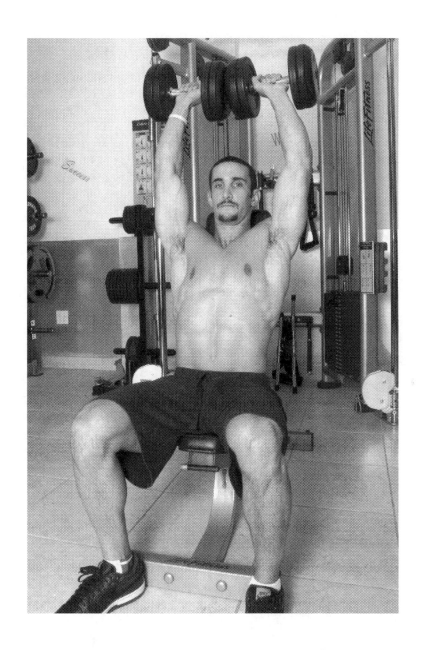

Arnold Presses – named after Arnold Schwarzenegger – place a great amount of stress on the front deltoid. I enjoy this exercise because it also works great for the side delts. It is a great exercise because it's the equivalent of super-setting (discussed later) DB presses with side lateral raises. This exercise can be performed either in a standing position or a seated position. Take one dumbbell in each hand and raise the weights to your shoulders with your palms facing you. From this point you begin to press the weights up overhead but not exactly the way you think. As you are pressing the weights up you are rotating your hands so that your palms are now going to face forward at the top of the movement. Once you complete the full range of motion start to reverse the movement by lowering the weights and rotating your hands back to the starting position. Make sure this is all done in a strict and control matter and do not make this a three part motion. In other words it should be done in a smooth natural motion.

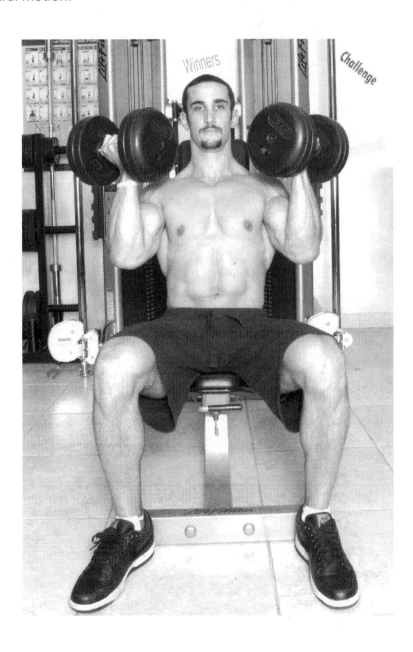

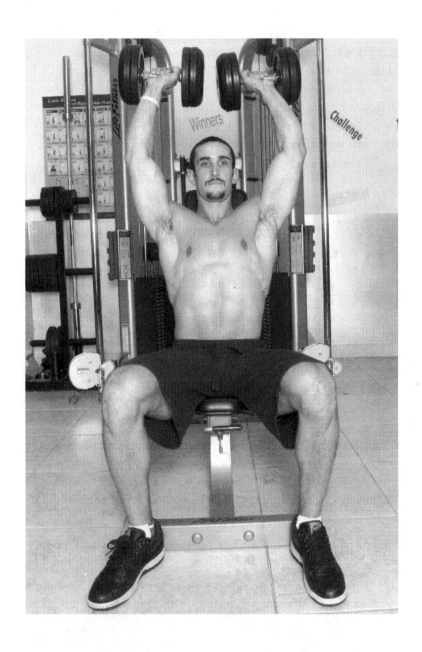

Front Raises – this particular exercise can be performed with dumbbells, barbell, cable attachments and even an e-z bar. Excellent form of exercise for maximum deltoid and chest separation. I enjoy using dumbbells until this day and I feel they allow me to get a better range of motion on the way up and on the way down. Stand or sit with a dumbbell in each hand and begin to lift one weight up in a controlled motion until it is higher than the top of your head. Lower the weight under control and begin to lift the other one in the same motion and repeat throughout each repetition. Make sure that you are using a comfortable weight so that way you don't use your body to cheat on the lifts. If you find yourself beginning to cheat and rock your knees then you can do one of three things: (1) use a lighter weight, (2) do them in a seated position for a stricter movement and (3) do them against a wall so that way your back is supported and cannot be used throughout the movement. To do this movement with either a barbell or straight bar cable attachment, simply grab the bar with an overhand grip and let it hang down at arm's length in front of your thighs. Once your grip is established begin to lift it in the same position like dumbbells – higher than your head and lower it in a controlled and strict fashion.

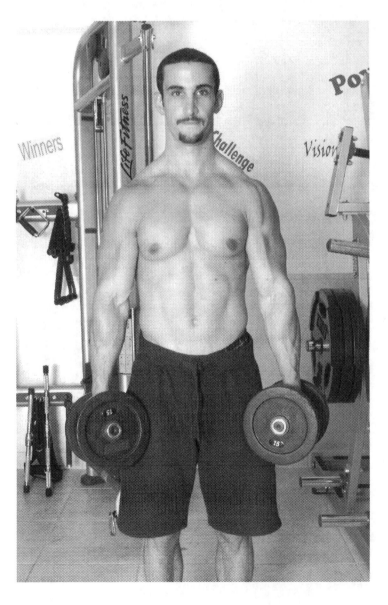

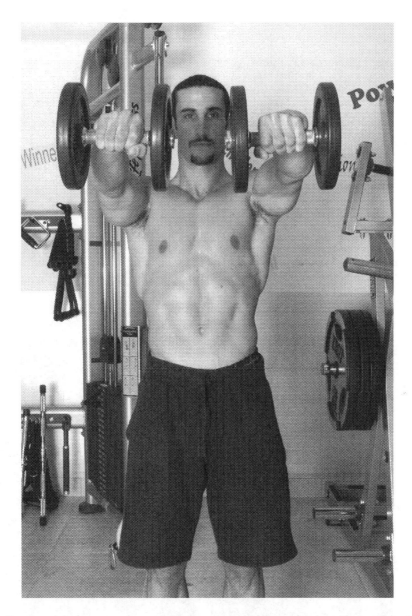

Dumbbells should always come as high as your chin or higher if possible. The only exception for this is when you go really heavy while trying to gain mass and size.

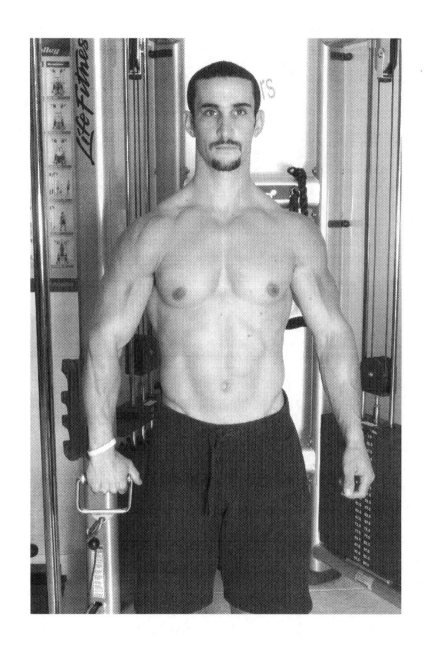

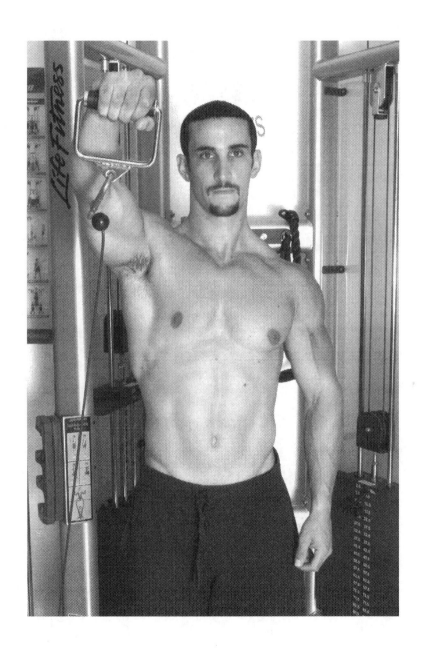

Incline DB Fly's – this is almost similar to chest fly's except for the fact that you are in a 75-90 degree position therefore placing more stress on the deltoids, yet still hitting the upper chest muscles. This exercise is not widely used and not many people even know what it is so no need to get too stressed out and ahead of ourselves. I like to do this exercise every so often to just get a burning sensation in my front deltoids.

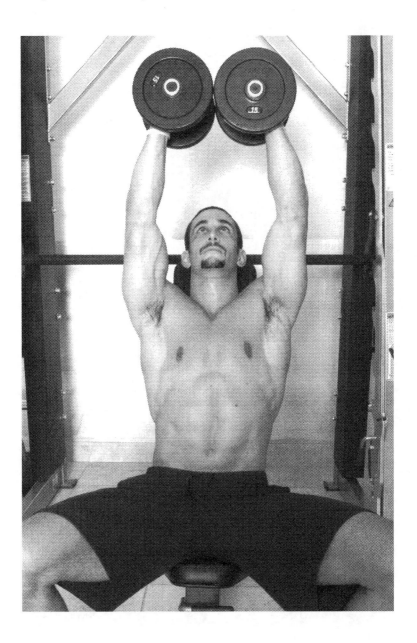

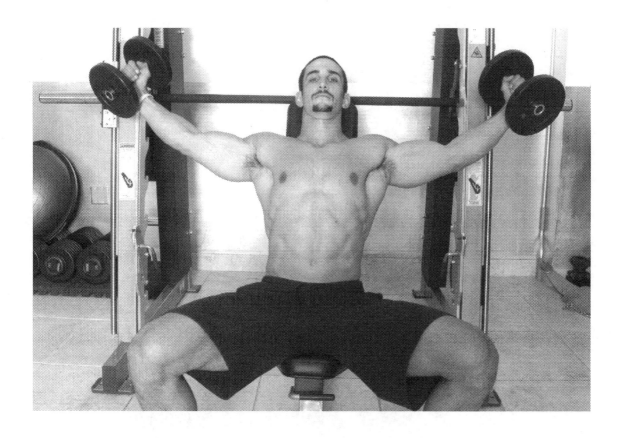

Side Deltoids (Lateral Deltoids)

Since most of the above related exercises hit this part of the deltoid there are not too many specific exercises for it. I do recommend, however, the following few exercises.

Side Dumbbell laterals – you can do this exercise either standing or seating. The difference between the two is that whenever you stand you tend to cheat a bit and use your knees or lower back as a way to lift the weights. On the contrary, a seated motion such as this exercise is hard to cheat on since your back is tightly up against the bench. I do see people cheat on this exercise by sitting closer to the edge of the bench. Thus, allowing them to rock back and forth and create momentum. If you want best results I recommend you do it strict, tight and correct. If you have to substitute weight for form then do it. In the long run you will have better developed deltoids and eventually can become a pro in the sense of form and control.

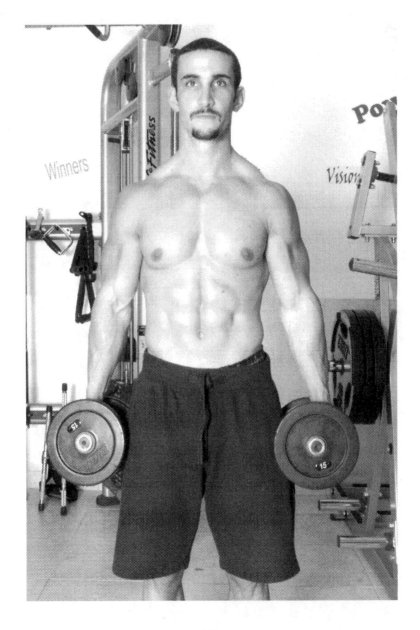

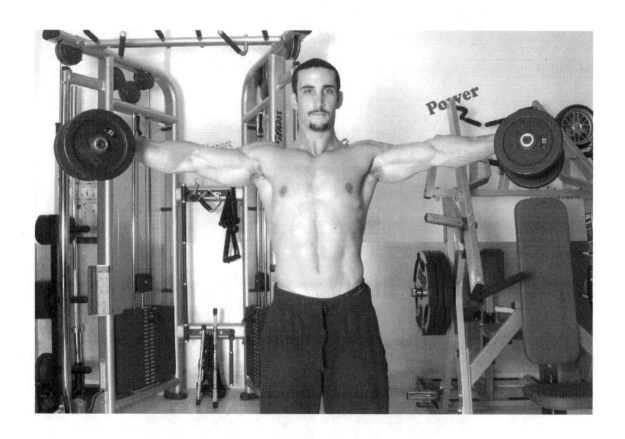

Cable Lateral Raises – same exercise as DB lateral raises just using a cable with a single grip handle. Since many pulley or cable machines work on resistance, this motion will feel harder and probably even a bit challenging. You really can't perform this exercise seated so while standing make sure that your knees are slightly bent and that they stay this way throughout the whole set. Do not jerk your knees or your back to create momentum and speed. This should be done in a strict manner and a controlled fashion. I love this exercise because I was able to see results almost immediately. My side deltoids got extremely striated and well defined.

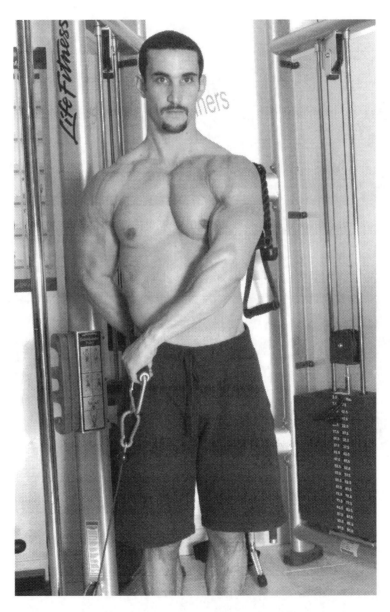

Notice that my wrist is bent a bit. You want to come up with the cable in a controlled fashion to fully execute the movement. Picture yourself pouring water from a pitcher as you begin to lower the weight. This is a demonstration of cable laterals from the front.

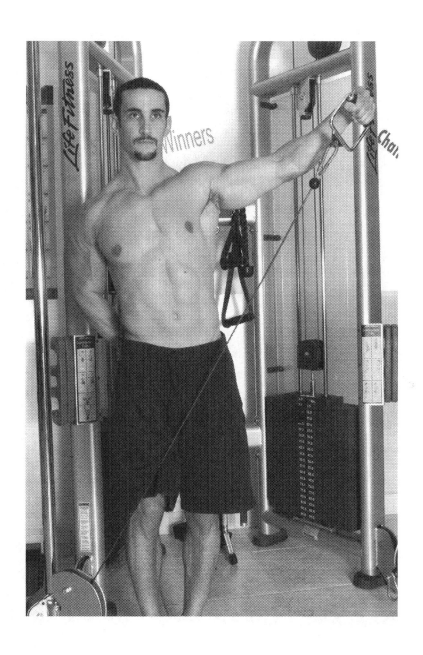

Here we see the same exercise but done to the back

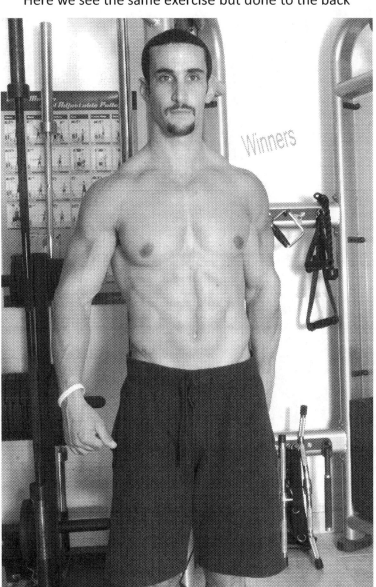

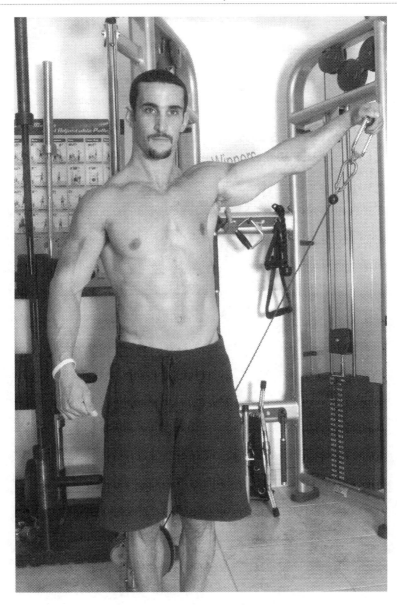

Burns after your Lateral Raises – what the hell is a burn? It is exactly what it sounds like – BURN. After you complete your sets for Lateral raises walk over to the dumbbell rack and take a fairly challenging weight. No need to be a hero and go all out because I have yet to explain what it is your going to do with these dumbbells. Now that you picked a moderate weight you hold them out to the side with totally straight arms approximately 12 to 15 inches from your thighs for as long as possible or for as long as it begins to BURN. Try to at least hold them up and out for 20-30 seconds.

Rear Deltoids (posterior delts)

Reverse Pec-Dec Fly's – same machine that you use for chest fly's except this time your face will be facing the machine. Make sure you keep your chest on the pad at all times. This is a good exercise to cool down after an intense shoulder routine and also a great way to begin an intense shoulder routine.

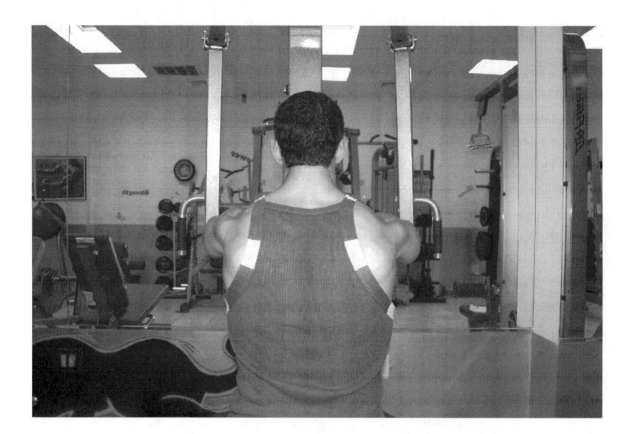

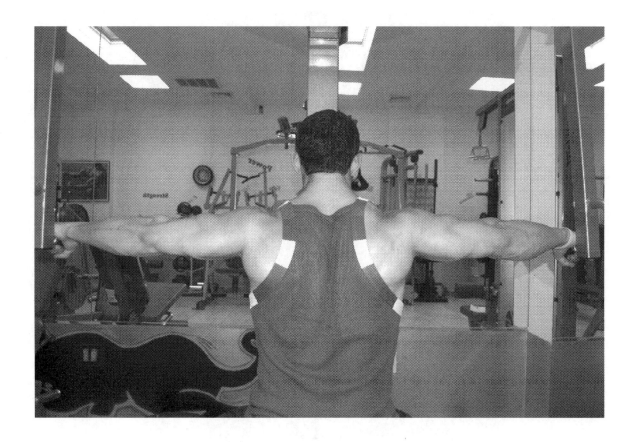

Seated Bent-Over Dumbbell Lateral Raises (great way to isolate the rear head of the deltoids (my absolute favorite). Sit on the edge of the bench with your knees together and a dumbbell in each hand. Bend forward from the waist and bring the dumbbells together behind your legs/calves with your palms facing each other. While keeping your body in control and steady lift the weights out to the side and pause for a second before lowering them again slowly to the starting position. Make sure that at all times your body is not lifting up and down and be sure that you are able to lift the dumbbells straight out to either side. Do not use your back or front deltoids to perform this exercise. In other words, DO NOT CHEAT DOING THIS EXERCISE.

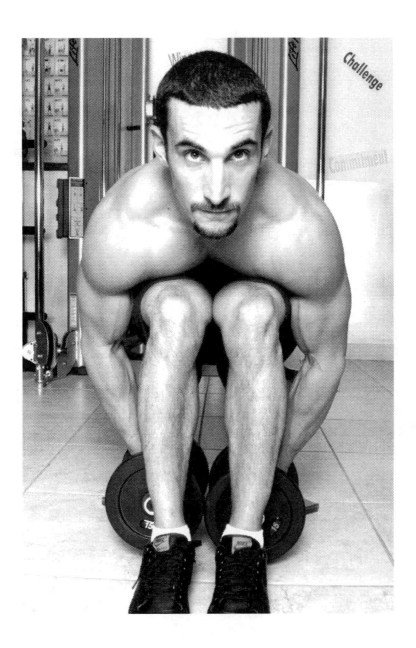

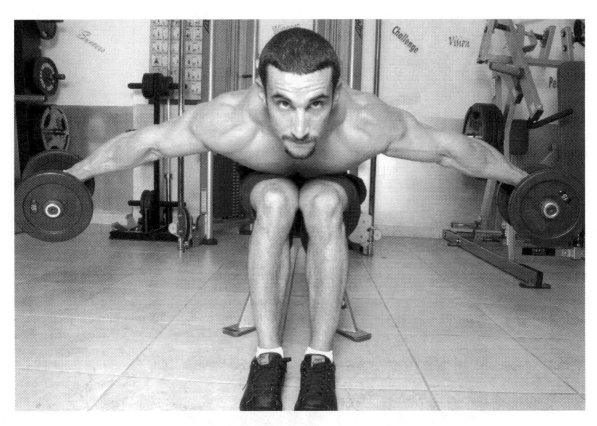

Make sure that your head is up at all times and your torso
right up against your thighs to ensure proper form.

Standing Bent-Over Dumbbell Lateral Raises – again the same exercise as above just not as strict as doing it seated. Stand with a dumbbell in each hand and bend forward from the waist about 45 degrees or more. Allow the dumbbells to hang at arm's length below you with your palms facing each other. Once you are positioned comfortably lift the weights out to either side of your head without raising or rocking your body. Lower the weights in a controlled resisting matter all the way down and repeat.

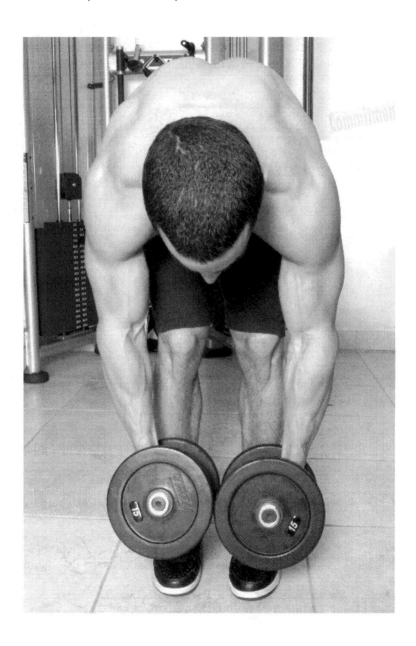

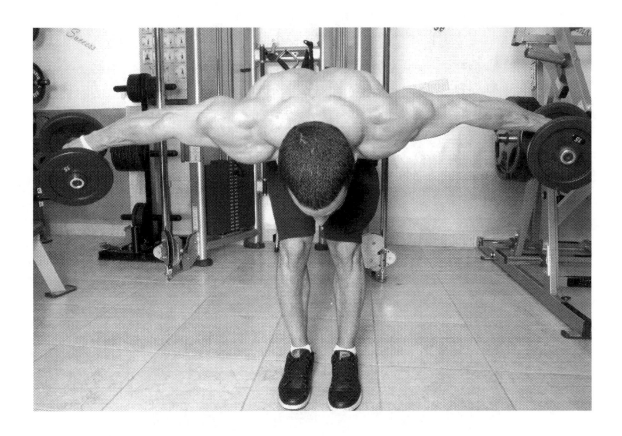

Bent-Over Cable Lateral's– by using the cables, you begin to get a longer range of motion with way more resistance then dumbbells throughout the movement. This exercise is performed by using two floor-level pulleys. Take a handle is each hand with your arms crossed in front of your body (left hand holding right side cable and right hand holding left side cable) and begin to bend down so that your torso is parallel to the floor. Pull smoothly bringing the handles across your body and extend your arms straight out to the sides. Arnold Schwarzenegger best described this procedure as turning your wrists slightly with your thumbs down as if you are pouring a pitcher of water. Once your arms are fully stretched then begin to release and let your arms come back slowly across your body as far in as they can.

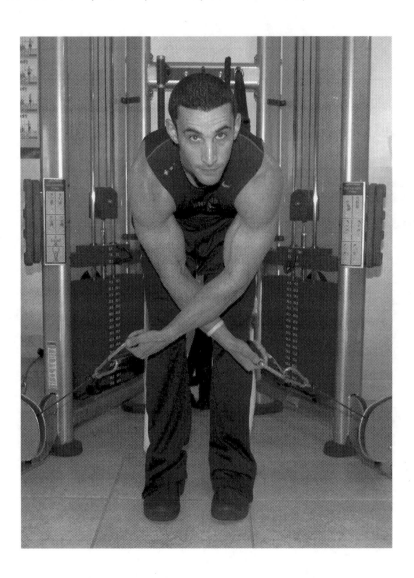

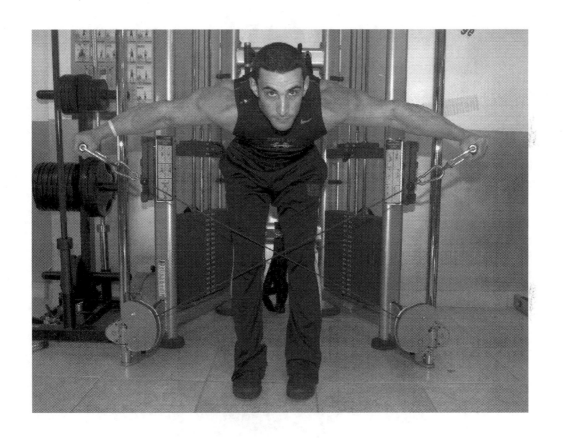

Trapezius

Upright Rows – you can use either a barbell, smith machine or cable bar attachment. Stand next to a barbell rack and grasp it with an overhand grip, keeping your hands about 8 to 10 inches apart. Let the bar hang straight down in front of you and lift it straight up until the bar reaches your chin. Make sure that the bar is kept close to your body at all times. Once the weight is up, lower it under control to the starting position and repeat. This exercise needs to be done in a strict and controlled form (absolutely no cheating or swinging the weight up). For variation you can use a short bar, cable straight bar or a fixated weighted barbell.

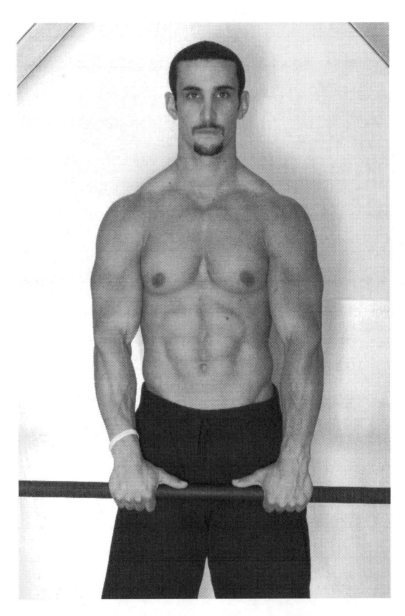

This is a close-grip position – you can change your hand positioning to a wider grip if more comfortable

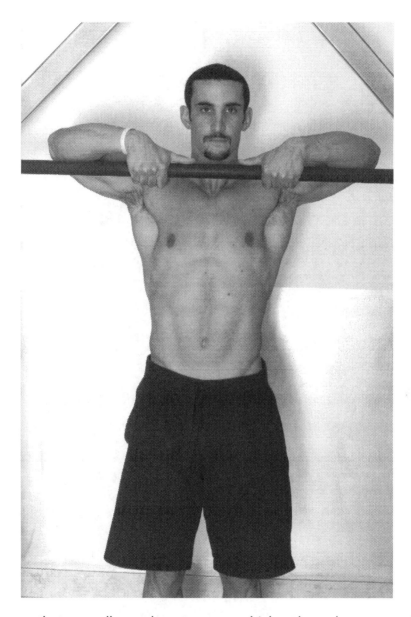

Make sure that your elbows do not come up higher than what you see in the picture. Your elbows and forearms should be almost parallel to the bar.

Barbell Shrugs or Smith Machine Shrugs – This exercise is done by holding a shoulder width grip. It can be performed either as an overhand grip or underhand grip. Both are extremely helpful in developing the trapezius muscle.

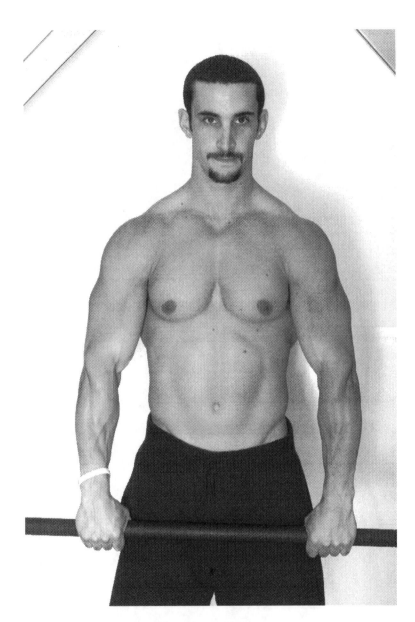

Smith Machine

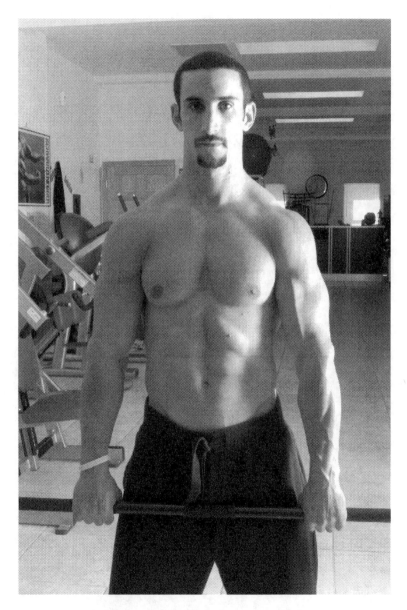

Barbell

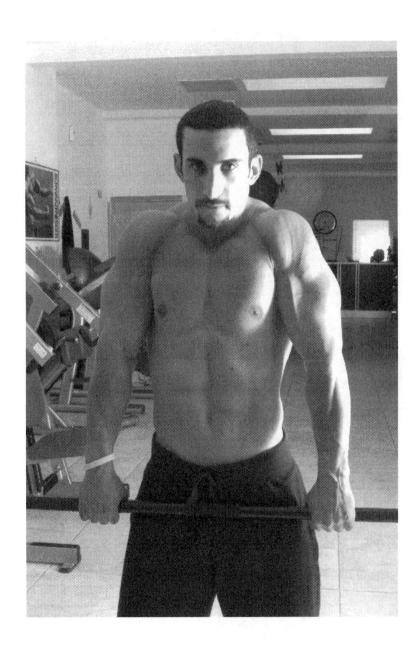

Dumbbell Shrugs – this allows you to increase the range of motion and contract the muscles a bit longer (Great for overall trapezius and back development). Stand upright with your arms at the sides holding a heavy dumbbell in each hand and raise your shoulders up as high as you can. The best way to get a full contraction is to attempt to reach your ears. Once you have lifted the dumbbells up hold for a second or two, then release and return to the starting position. Make sure that you are using strict form and not moving anything but your shoulders.

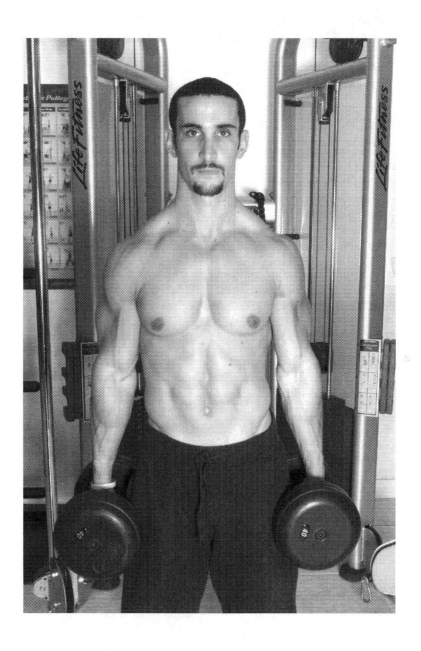

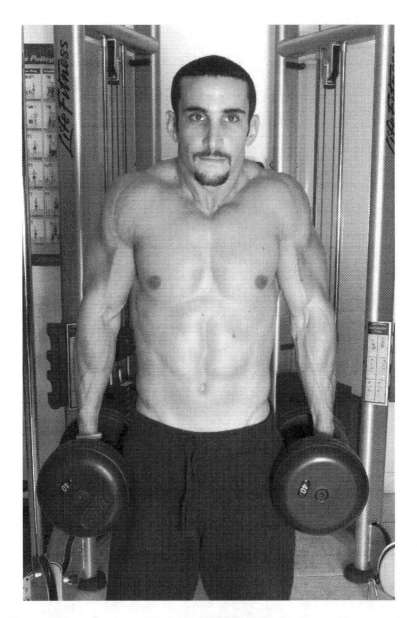

The only muscle that should be working is your trapezius muscle.
No arms, legs or any other bodypart should be involved.

Chapter 6
Peaks – Working Your Arms

This is the chapter that many will read over and over again for the simple fact that everyone relates to the arms. Wow how big are your arms? What exercises do you do to see results? How did you get that ball looking muscle? These are common everyday questions that I hear often and I am sure that there are so many others. The arms consist of three major muscle groups: The **Biceps Brachii**, a two-headed muscle that allows to lift and curl the arm, the **Triceps Brachii,** a three-headed muscle that works in opposition to the biceps and the **Forearm,** the muscles by the wrist and up to the elbow. As a kid growing up I was totally impressed with big bulging arms especially in Schwarzenegger's films. How were they so big? And at the same time how was he agile? They reminded me of mountain peaks that never seemed to end. They were absolutely a great sight and I am sure I was not the only one who thought so. I use to go through numerous magazines and publications as I began to bodybuild looking for examples and photos of outstanding arms and promised myself that I would one day have nice developed and well shaped arms. Since the arms are considered a small muscle the amount of exercises are great in numbers. There are so many different positions and angles to work with. I still see new exercises at local gyms as well as new people experimenting to create the best arm exercise. There are certain exercises that target the arms and help develop them tremendously. On the other hand, as I always say, do what you think best works for you. You know your body better than anyone. You can try to do what the big guy across the gym is doing but just know that if it works for him it might not work for you. Be open-minded, experimental and decipher what you think works best for YOU. You can develop perfect arms with hard work and proper training techniques but you must also take into consideration your genes and their potential. Everyone is shaped differently and has different bone and density structure. Thank God for that, otherwise we will all be walking around with huge round peaked biceps. There are many different shaped biceps to accommodate almost every body type whether you're short, tall, average, etc...

Each person must find their strengths and weaknesses and work to achieve perfection. Try to use variety and exercises that only require the use of biceps. It is very easy to use other muscles or stabilizers while performing bicep exercises such as curls. Try to totally isolate this small two-headed muscle and direct all the tension and weight on it rather than let's say on your shoulders or back. Be smart and use good judgment while doing a session of biceps. Concentrate on the motion, contract hard and picture your biceps the way you want them to look. This sounds a bit hard to grasp but I can guarantee that once you try it, your arms will begin to take shape. Remember, working out is a vision, it's a journey that you embarked on for some reason. If you dream it, then why not have it. Be assertive, positive, dedicated and know your goal for I assure you everything else will fall into place.

Part I - BIG BOY ARMS (Bicep's Training)

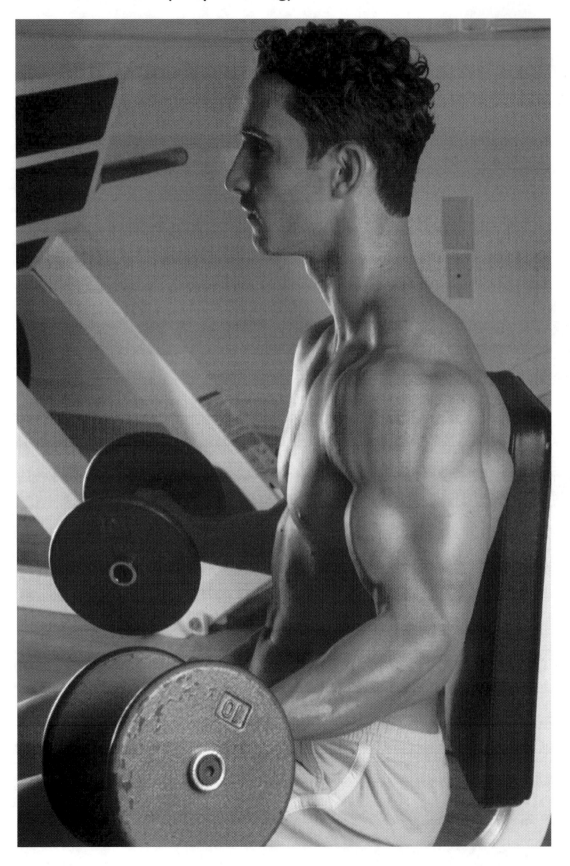

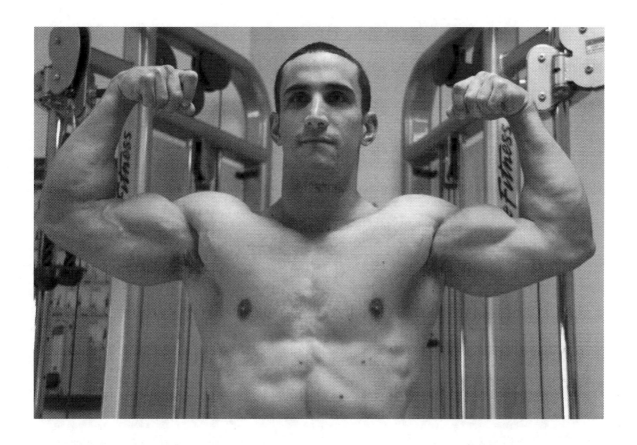

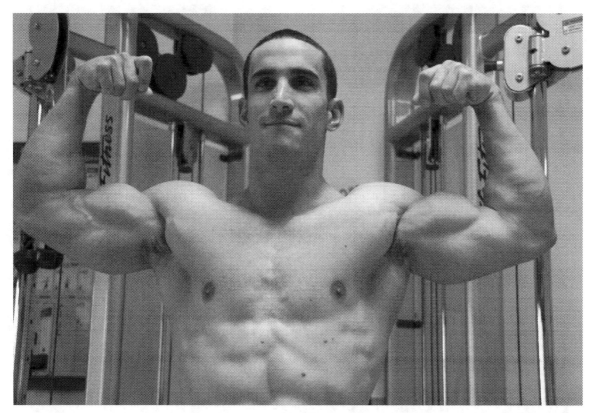

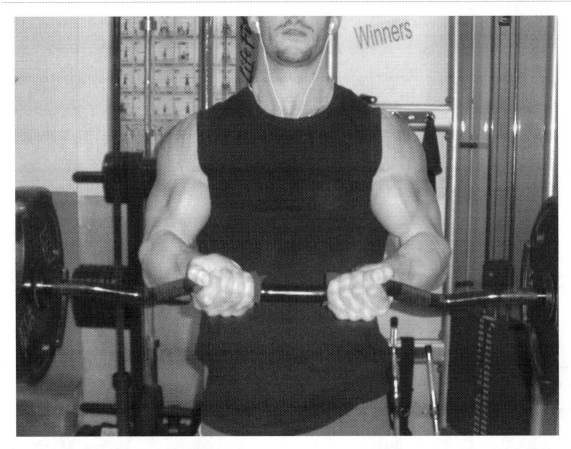

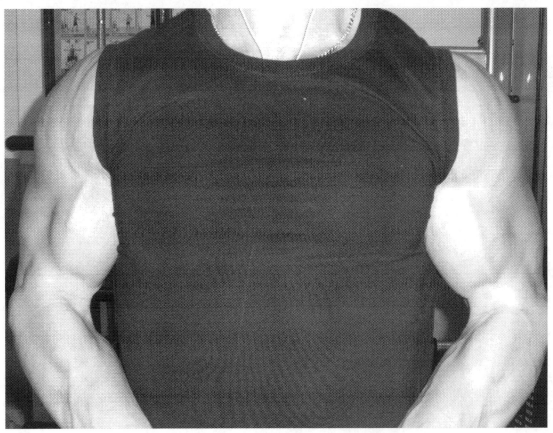

For mass and overall thickness you must begin to customize heavy compound movements that stress both heads of the biceps. Muscle size comes from lifting heavy weights. Your repetitions should be around 6 to 8 and you must visualize your arms as growing to BIG ARMS status. The exercises listed below are the most popular and the most portrayed exercises in many fitness magazines.

Barbell Curls – you can hold either a shoulder width grip or a close grip – both grips work very well and place a great stress of tension on the heads of the biceps. Begin by standing upright with your elbows at sides and arms fully extended. This extension of the arms allows the biceps to fully stretch. Start to curl the bar out and up as high as you can while keeping your elbows close to your body at all times. Make sure to fully flex and contract the bicep at the end of the movement before lowering to the start position. In addition, make sure that your form is strict and that you are not using any body movement as a means to lift the weight.

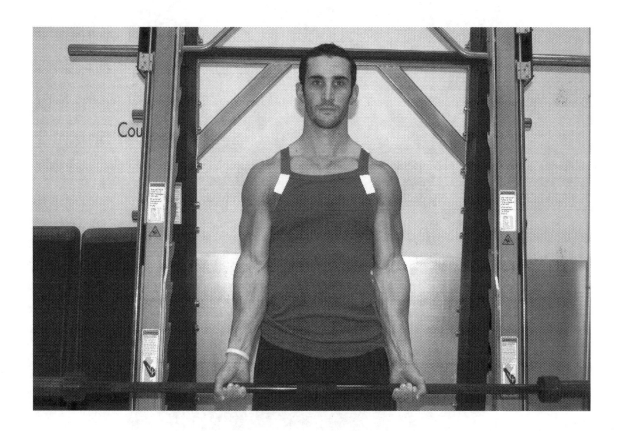

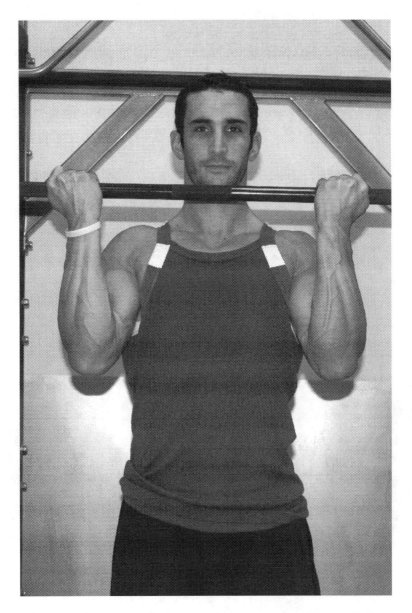

Make sure that your elbows are close to your sides at all times.

Alternate DB Curls – this exercise can either be performed standing or seated as long as you don't cheat and get a full controlled range of motion. A very common exercise amongst bodybuilders and is at times considered the "meat and potatoes" of biceps. Stand upright with a dumbbell in each hand hanging at arm's length. Curl one dumbbell forward and up as high as you can while flexing the bicep throughout. Then bring it back down under control through the same motion and begin to curl the other hand up. Be sure to keep your elbows steady and tight on your side or waist. You can also do alternate dumbbell curls in a sitting position and even curl both hands up simultaneously.

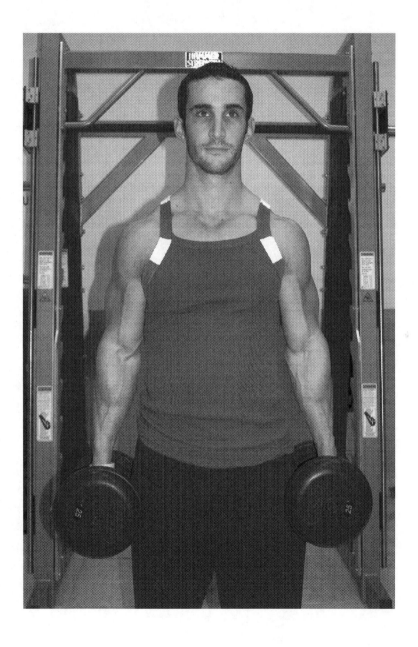

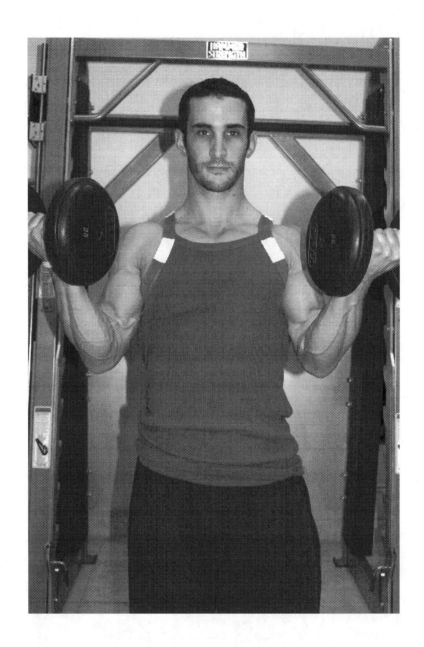

21's – this exercise is mostly used to shape and develop the entire biceps muscle. It is also a great exercise to test your endurance levels – 21's refer to 3 parts and each part consists of 7 repetitions. There is a half curl, a cheat curl and a full range of motion curl. No matter if you're a beginner or a professional everyone feels this exercise the same. The burn is immense and just a great exercise to add to your itinerary. You can perform this exercise with a barbell, dumbbells and cable bar attachments (straight bar, wide-grip bar, e-z bar).

Part One
Seven Repetitions
Half Curl

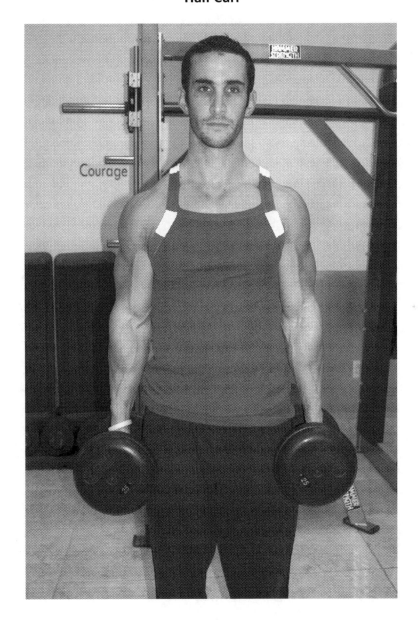

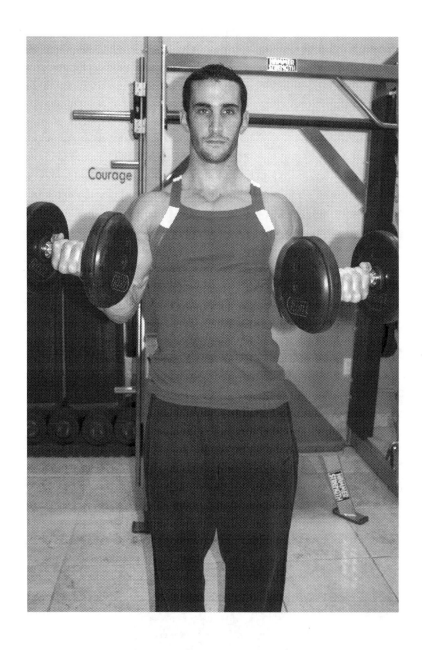

Part Two
Seven Repetitions
Cheat Curls

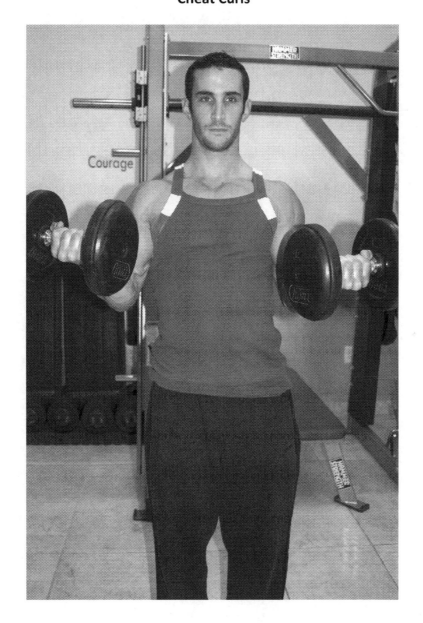

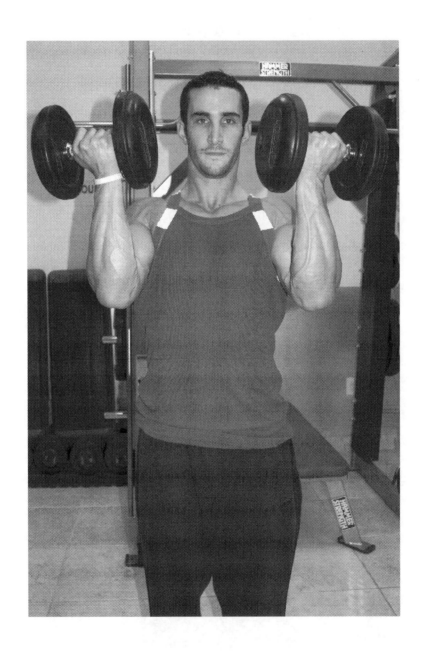

Part Three
Seven Repetitions
Full Curls

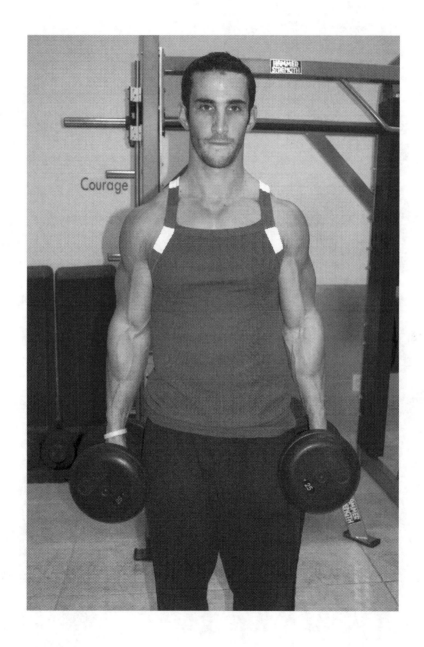

Spider Curls – make sure you use a heavy weight that can be used for 6-8 reps. This exercise is done on an adjustable bench. Make sure that the bench is positioned to 90 degrees to ensure proper and adequate tension.

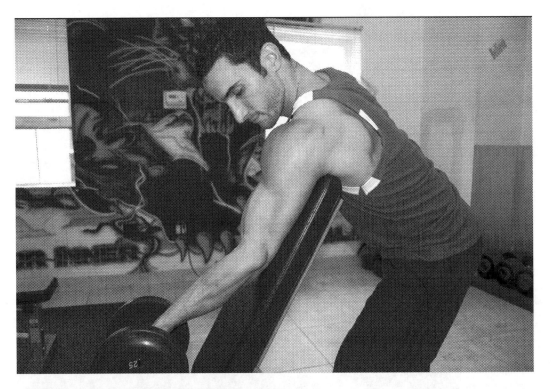

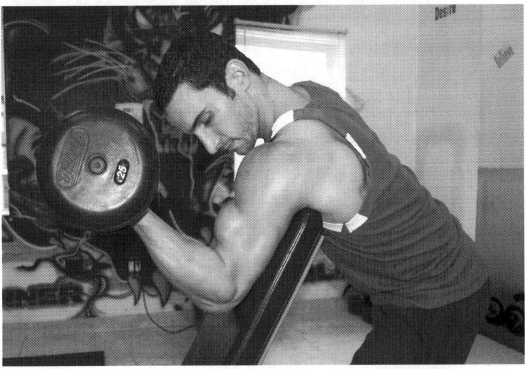

To ensure proper form make sure that your armpit is locked on top of the bench. This will place a great amount of stress on the bicep.

Thickness in the biceps is vital but height is also another common overlooked factor. If you want your biceps to stand out and get noticed then start trying to work on its peak or height. You should perform exercises such as:

Concentration Curls with a dumbbell or cable (mostly always done with a dumbbell and make sure your form is perfect to ensure results). This exercise is great for targeting your biceps in an isolation movement. Hold a dumbbell in one arm and sit on the edge of a bench or chair with your feet a few inches apart. Lean a tad bit forward from your hips and place the elbow against the inside of your thigh. Allow the dumbbell to hang down at arm's length with your palm facing the other leg and begin to curl the dumbbell almost up to your shoulder. Make sure to keep strict form throughout the exercise and at no times bend too far forward or too far back as a way to lift the weight (that's cheating).

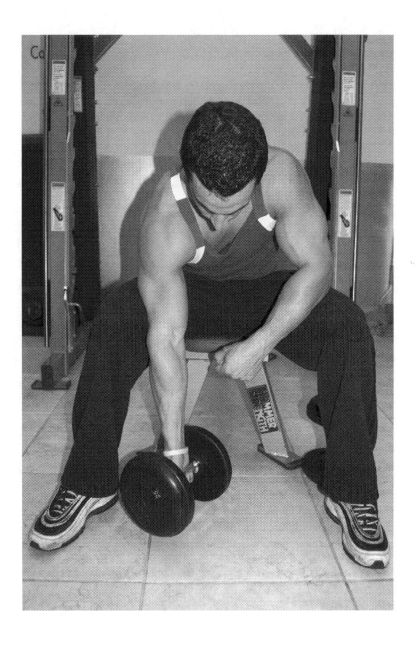

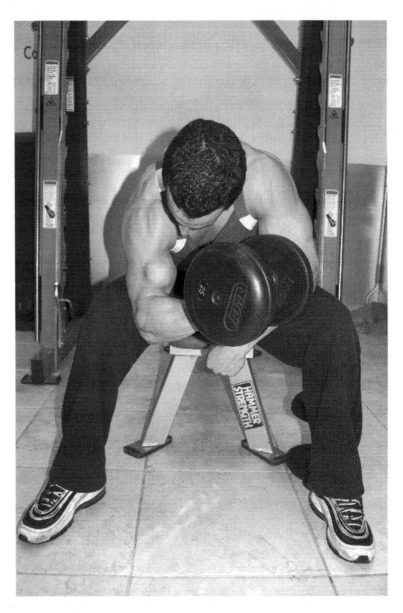

OR

You can also do concentration curls in a hammer curl fashion. Same as regular concentration curls except for a slight different angle in the form. Here is an example:

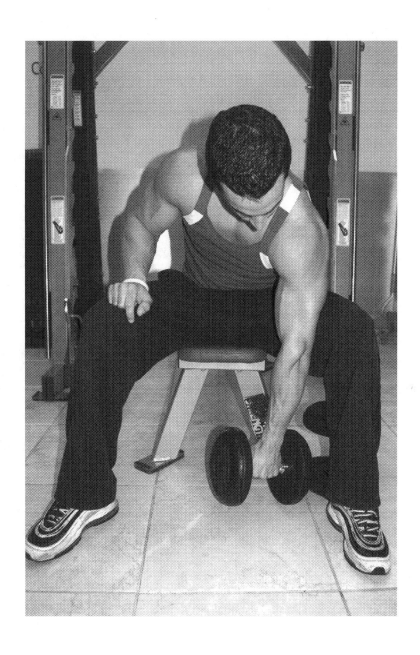

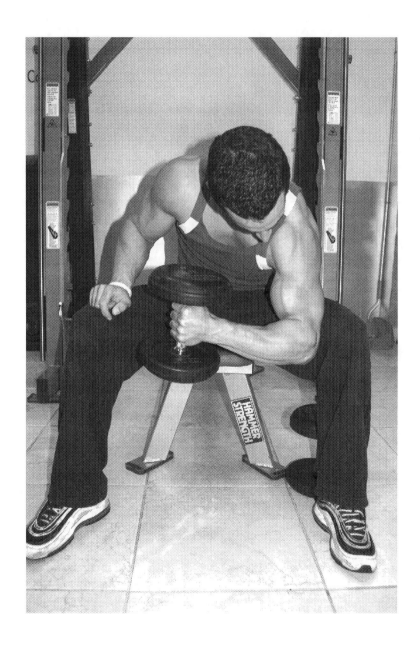

Cable Curls – this exercise should be done while using the contraction principle. This principle involves flexing of the biceps as hard as possible at the end of the movement allowing for an extreme contraction. Almost like flexing hard and holding that pose for a few seconds.

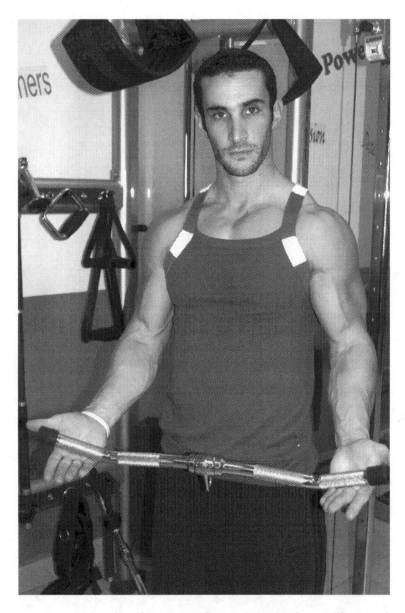

Here is an example of wide-grip curls using an e-z bar cable attachment

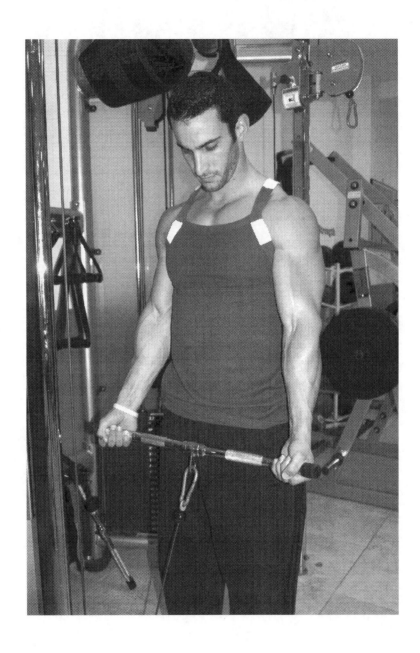

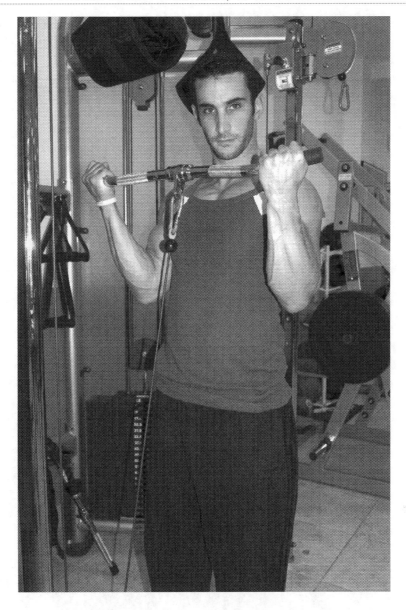

In addition to these exercises you can do many other curls using dumbbells or machines and doing it to failure or till you get a tremendous pump. This pump, or an accumulation of blood rushing to that area, will aid greatly in achieving height in the biceps.

For outer Thickness and definition (This is known as the outer head, the one facing away from the armpit)

Barbell Curls – inward or close grip. Both are effective and just becomes a matter of how much pressure the wrists can handle.

Preacher Curls – close grip handle position or even dumbbells. The dumbbells allow each arm to work independently and develop strength. Make sure your movement when using dumbbells is stable, controlled, and strict. Preacher curls are truly a strict movement and place so much tension on the biceps. Position yourself with your chest against the bench/

pad with your arms extending over it. I like to tell my clients that to ensure proper form their armpits have to be locked under the padding of the preacher bench. Take hold of the barbell or e-z bar with an underhand grip. Making sure your body is straight and steady, curl the bar all the way up and then lower it again to its full extension. Make sure your elbows are close together and at no time flaring out. This will ensure proper tension, stress and contraction on the biceps.

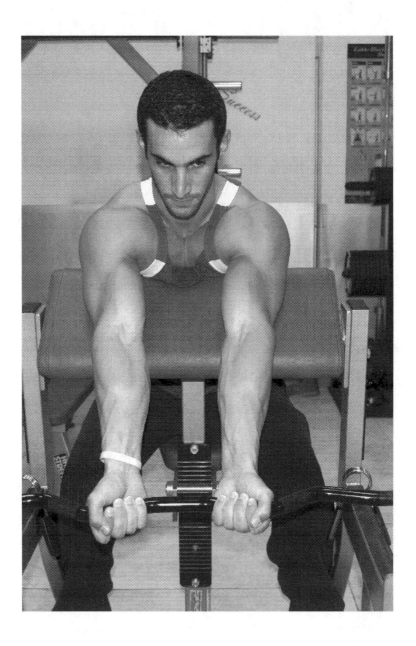

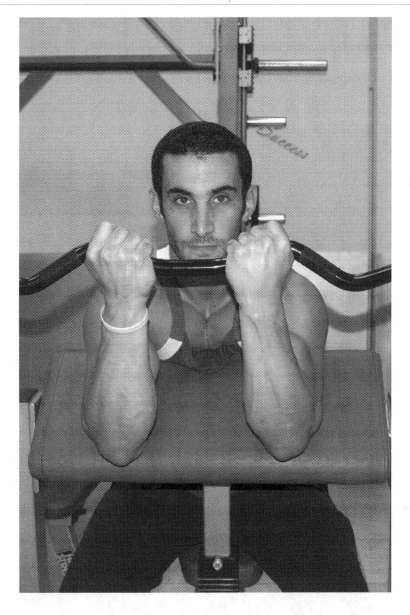

Cable Curls – close grip: Once again depending how much pressure your wrists can endure you can modify the exercise and move your wrists up to eight inches apart and still maintain a fairly close grip.

For inner Thickness and definition (this is known as the inner head, the one facing the armpit) your hand position should be shoulder width apart or even wider if your wrists do not hurt).

Standing Barbell Curls- Do not work on momentum. Ensure strict form throughout each rep and set.

Preacher Curls with either an e-z bar or a barbell

Dumbbell Hammer Curls – This exercise is great for both the biceps and the forearms. It is done the same way as regular dumbbells curls except for the fact that the palms face inward and stay that way throughout the movement. This exercise can be done either standing or sitting.

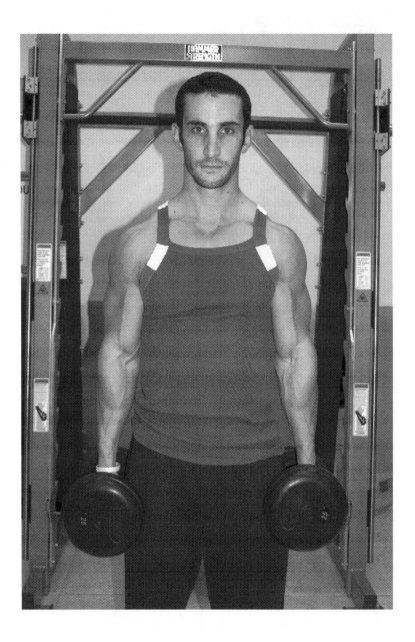

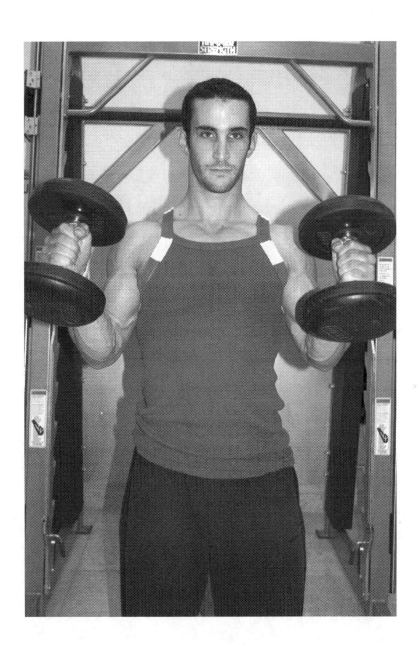

OR

You can do hammer curls using a rope cable attachment

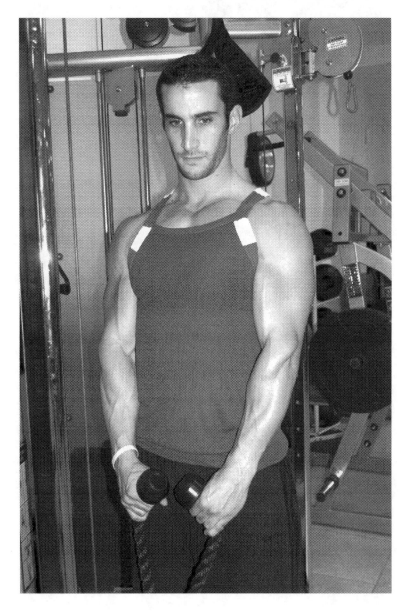

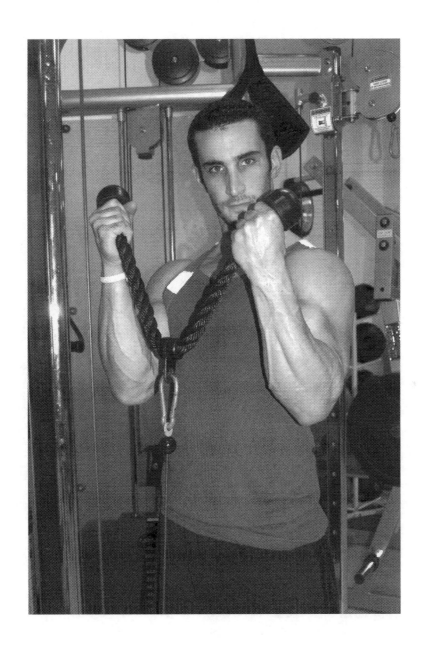

Incline Dumbbell Curls – great exercise for stretching the biceps and overall development. Sit back on an incline bench holding a dumbbell (a manageable weight) in each hand. Making sure that your back is against the bench and your elbows forward throughout the movement, curl the weights forward and up to shoulder level. Once the dumbbells are up, begin to contract for a second before lowering the weights again fully under control. Make sure to never use any momentum by swinging the weights on this exercise.

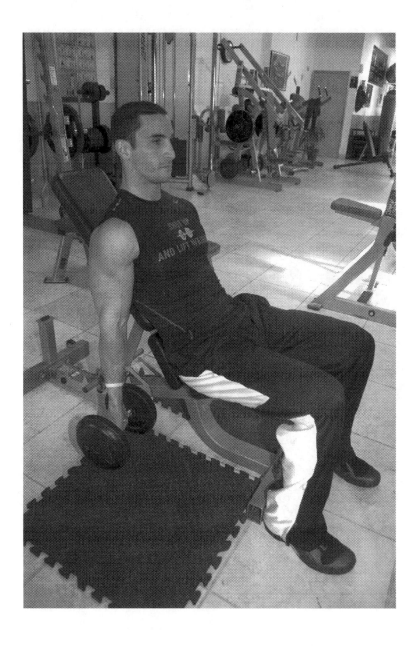

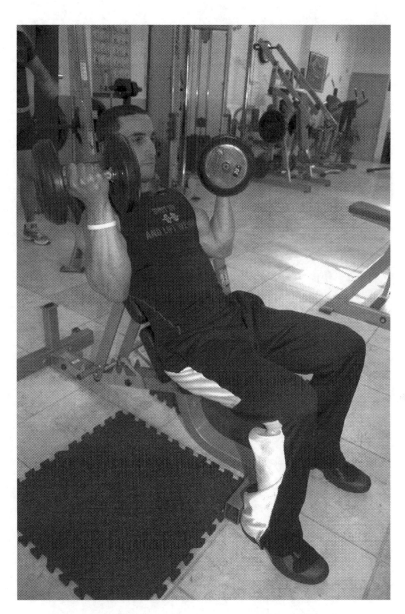

Make sure that you get a full range of motion while keeping your elbows at your side at all times.

Incline Hammer Dumbbell Curls – same exercise as regular incline dumbbell curls with the exception of your palms facing inward. Maintain strict form and control throughout the movement.

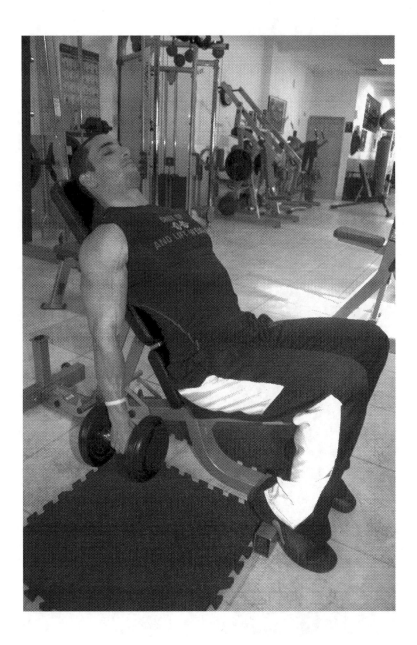

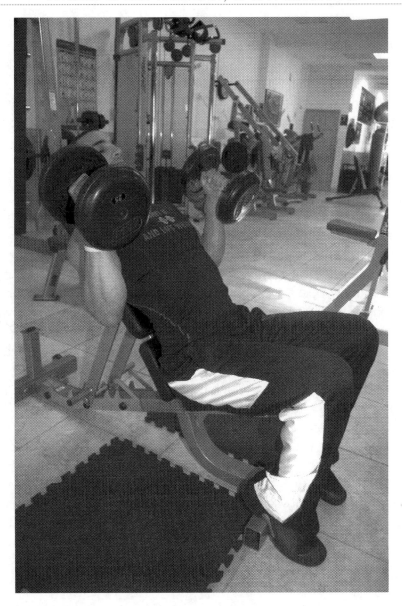

I cannot stress how important proper technique is required in achieving those peaked biceps you wanted. Review these four rules so that next time you work out biceps you will feel better and actually even begin to see results:

- Variety – switch around your routines using dumbbells, barbells, cables and machines

- Isolation – don't get help from the deltoids, lower back or other body parts when training biceps. Don't swing the weight or work on momentum (in other words, if you cheat than its too heavy)

- Full range of motion – as this implies, move the weight in a groove – locate the natural line of motion for each repetition and each movement to get maximum results

- Total concentration – all your distractions have to be placed on the side when training biceps. Don't let your mind wander; always stay fixated on the movement and the feeling in the muscle

In case I forgot to mention, ideally the size of your bicep should resemble the size of your calf. I thought this piece of information will be an inspiration to start working out both your calf and bicep muscles.

Part II – TRI ME (working the triceps')

The triceps are a bit more complicated in a sense that there are three different heads to execute. I recommend that all your tricep exercises be done strictly and in perfect form. Try to really get a good contraction allowing the muscle to fully extend and flex. Keep your elbows at your side the whole time while using any type of cable and cable attachment. You absolutely want to totally flex your triceps throughout the entire motion. Once again, I can't overemphasize how important strict form is on the exercises of this three-headed muscle. Just imagine, in only a few sets you will begin to feel a burn and a sick pump. All that lactic acid in that area is going to make your arms feel great. Almost as great as when you actually start taking notice that your arms (biceps and triceps) now have some sort of definition. I love it when my clients come over to me and begin to roll up their sleeves and show me that their arms are now beginning to pop out. They tell me, amongst other things, "I can't believe how they now look as compared to a few months ago." Everyone I know takes their arms for granted but I can assure you once you develop a bit of strength you will never make that mistake again.

For overall mass and thickness I suggest you use some heavy weight and make sure you are getting a full contraction. Try to place most of the stress on the triceps rather than your chest or shoulders. Here are some exercises that should be of great use:

Close-Grip Barbell Presses – either can be done with a smith machine or a bench press station (previously mentioned)

Overhead Dumbbell Extension – great exercise since the dumbbell allows you to get a good range of motion. In most cases with tricep exercises you want to lock your elbows at the top of the movement assuring great tension and peak contractions. If you are doing this movement standing then bend your knees a drop and try not to over-work your back. If you are seated while doing this exercise then make sure that the bench you are using can support your lower back and allow you to get a proper range of motion.

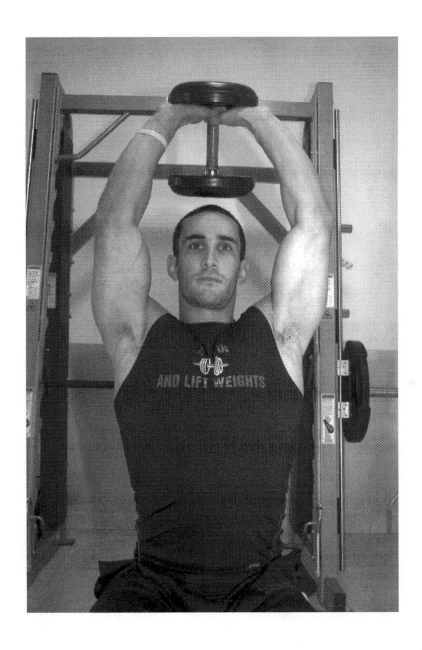

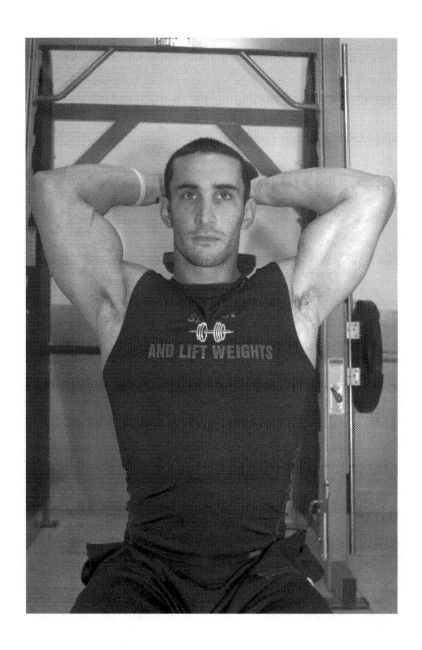

Dips – these can be done either with weight added using a belt of some sort or without. Both are effective and place great stress on all three heads of the triceps.

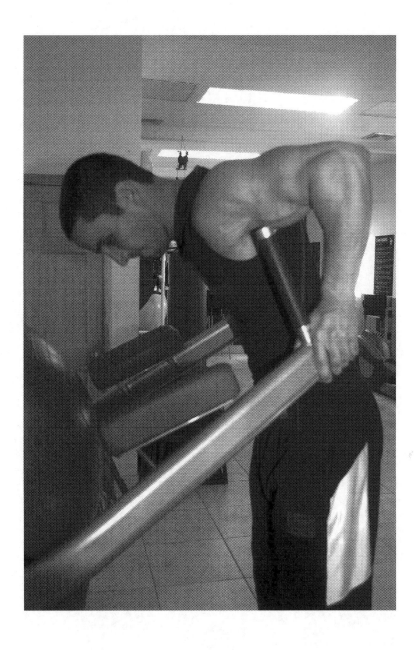

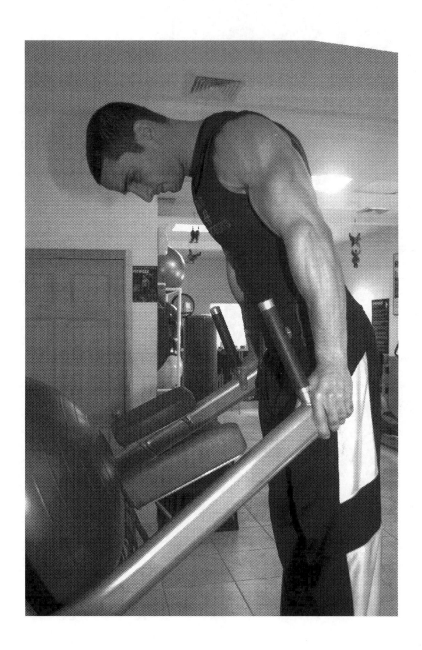

Heavy Kickbacks (using a dumbbell) - Make sure your elbows are at your side the whole time. Start this exercise by standing with your knees bent and one foot in front of the other as a form of balance. Take a dumbbell in one hand, bend your arm and raise your elbow back and up to about shoulder height. Keeping your elbow stationary, begin to press the weight back until your forearm is parallel to the floor and hold there for a moment to ensure maximum contraction before slowly coming back to the starting position.

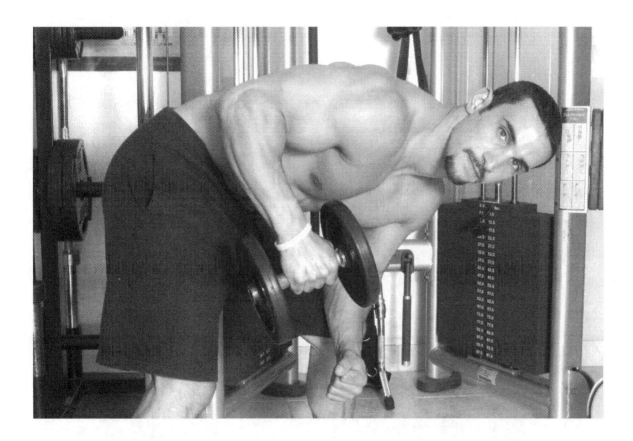

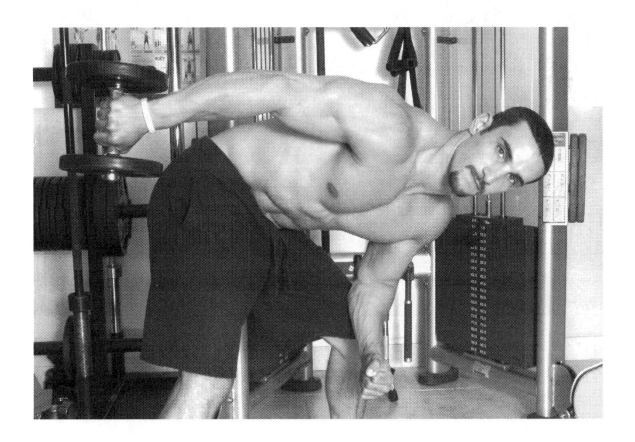

Skull-Crushers or French-Press – this exercise is done mostly with an e-z bar curl because it tends to be easier on the wrists for many, including myself. However, some people do it with a straight bar or even a pair of dumbbells. No right or wrong way of doing it; just depends on preference. This is usually done lying on a flat bench. It is done by raising the bar directly over your shoulders while both feet are on the ground. Keeping your arms still and above, make sure your elbows are kept in and not flaring out while lowering the bar to your forehead. Now it's called a skull-crusher because along the way you will hit your head and get a bruise, but no big deal. I hit my head plenty of times and I am well, or at least I think I am. Just a side note, this exercise tends to put a great deal of stress on the elbows so changing every once in a while from your routine is recommended. I use to do this exercise extremely heavy and often and within a year or two I was beginning to have severe elbow and joint problems. I later found out that I had severe tennis elbow or a form of tendonitis.

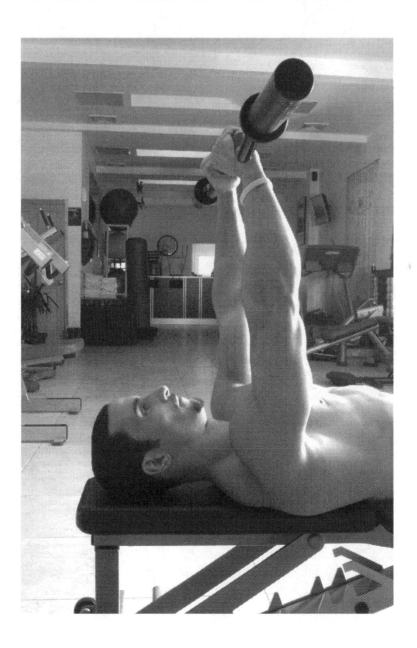

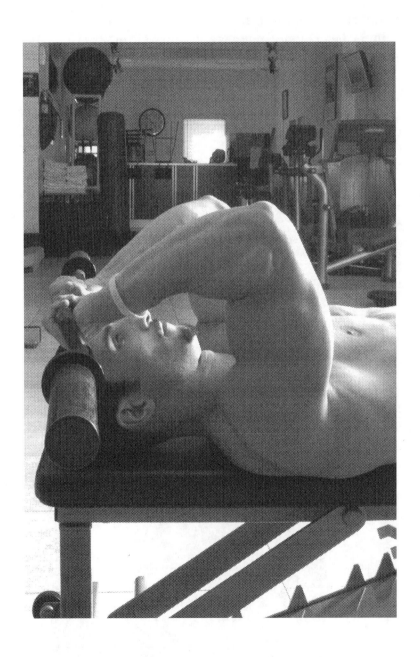

Or

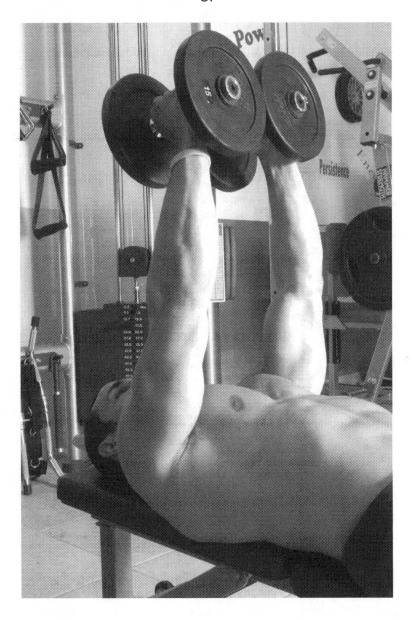

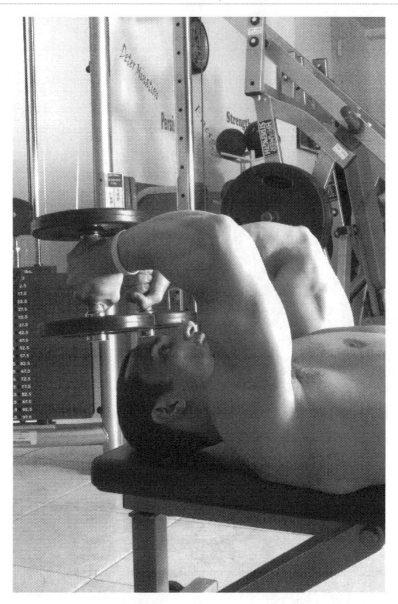

The above mentioned exercises are great for overall mass and thickness. However, there is a great deal of exercises that I will now mention for the other sections of the triceps. Same rules pretty much apply for these exercises – lock your elbows, keep proper strict form and always try to get a maximum contraction. Another good way to get a burn is by simply doing a few sets of a certain exercise 15-20 repetitions at a moderate weight and only resting 15 seconds. This will create a great pump and a huge amount of lactic acid in the triceps.

Cable Press downs - remember I went over many of the cable attachments in a previous chapter? Well this muscle needs a good variety of attachments to shock it and gain progress. V-bar, e-z bar, straight bar, rope, single-grip and a few others should suffice. Now don't go and do every single attachment you can find for four sets with high repetitions. The journal you are using should better aid you in terms of what you have done on previous workouts. It is important to change frequently, but remember if something works for you then stick with it. Many clients I have trained feel comfortable with a certain cable attachment for whatever reason they have. Maybe it's comfortable on their wrists, maybe they see results using this attachment, maybe they read many articles telling them to use a certain attachment and the list goes on and on. If you feel comfortable using an attachment of some sort then just use it and don't settle for an explanation from your trainer. You can listen and maybe even try but at the end you are your best critic. "If it ain't broke, then don't fix it."

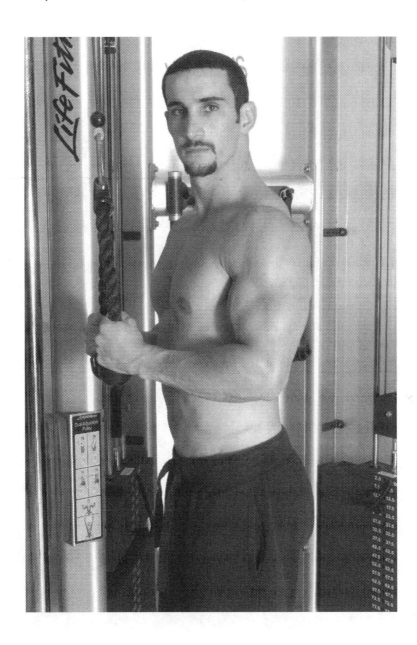

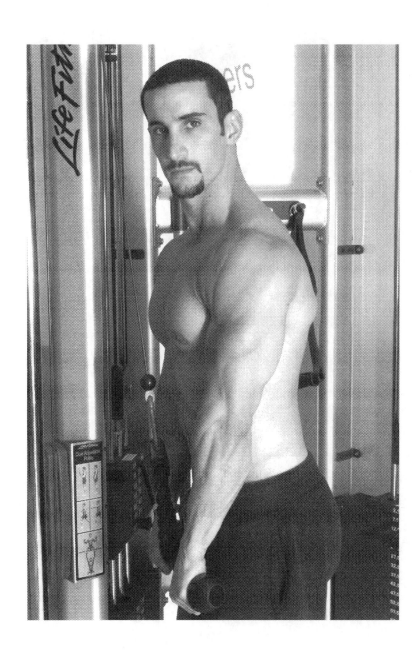

Overhead Cable Extension – this is similar to the overhead DB extension except for the fact that you are standing on this exercise and using a controlled weight and a cable attachment. Great exercise for developing the back-head of your triceps (the head closest to your armpit). Once again make sure your elbows are close together and not flaring out.

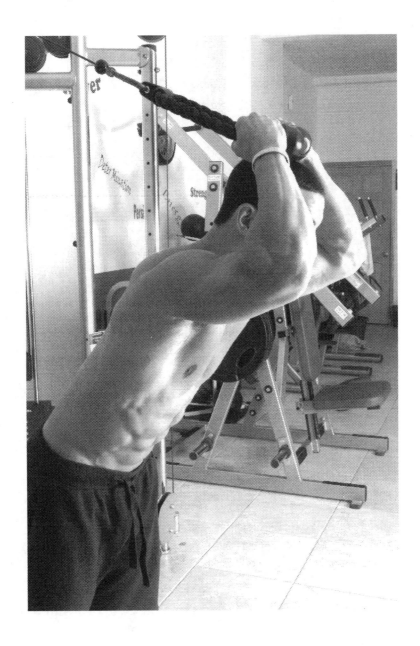

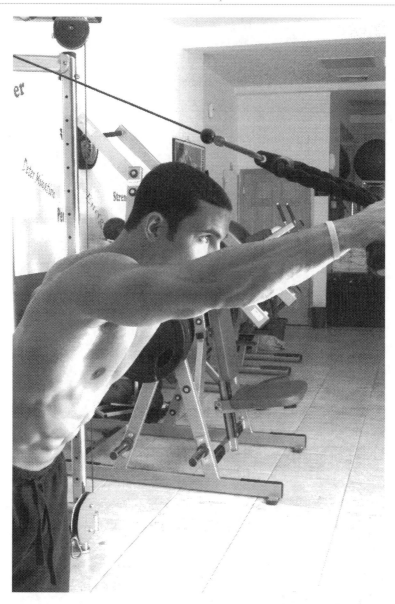

Make sure you get a full extension and a good contraction. Remember, you can use any cable attachment for this exercise (v-bar, straight bar, rope, etc...)

Bench Dip – you can perform this exercise either using one bench or using two benches. If you are using a single bench then make sure you sit on the edge of it with your legs together and straight in front of you. Place your hands about 6 to 8 inches apart holding it in a reverse fashion while griping the edge of the bench. Slide your butt off the bench slowly and begin to push yourself up. Once the elbows are locked you are in a contracting position so continue to lower yourself down and repeat. Your back and butt should always be close to the bench, almost as if they are grazing it. This will allow the movement to be strict and in no means do you thrust yourself up – meaning that your hips don't move. Only your elbows are moving. The wider you go out with your feet, the harder the motion becomes and vice versa. If you're a beginner, rather than extending your legs totally out in front of you, bend your knees to the angle you feel most comfortable in. Like I said, once you develop good form, your strength will increase and in no time will you be doing bench dips with your feet totally out in front of you. Now in the case of using two benches, the rules are almost the same except for the positioning of your feet. While with one bench you are gripping the bench and keeping your feet on the floor. With two benches your body is now in mid air, meaning that your butt is on the edge of one bench while your feet are on the edge of the second bench. The movement is the same but this exercise is a bit more challenging because it allows for a greater range of motion. In addition, if you are working out with a partner you can have them place weighted plates on your legs (above the knees and centered) for a tougher and more challenging movement. In my days of heavy lifting and competing I use to have my training partner stack at least four to five 45 pound plates on my body. Wow did it burn, especially while drop setting every plate.

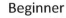

Beginner

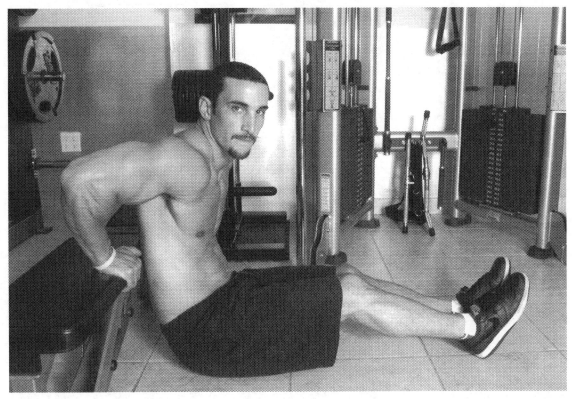

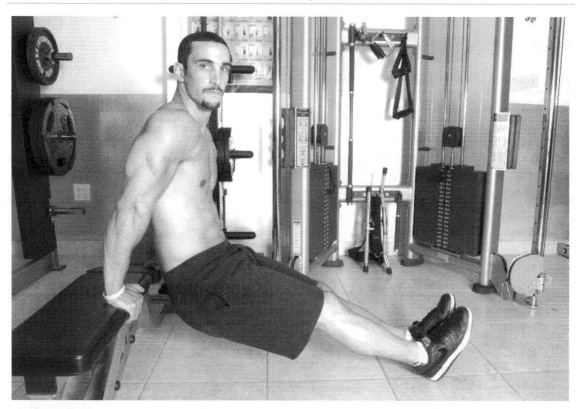

Advanced

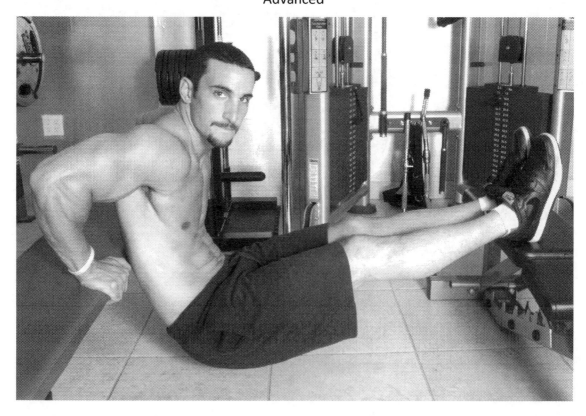

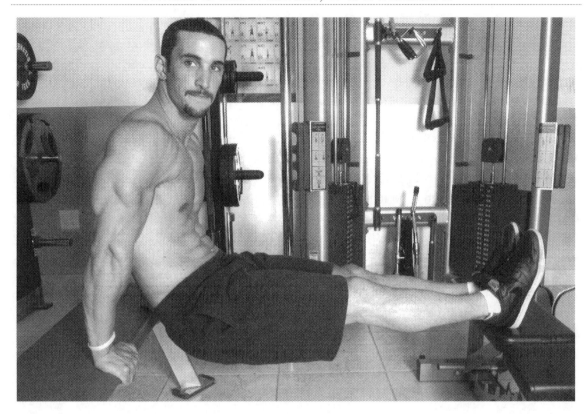

Close-grip or Diamond Push-up's – always a great way to finish up your arm routine. Just do one set to failure after you complete your tricep workout and you will see the burn you get from these push-up's.

One-Arm Overhead DB extension – this exercise is a crowd pleasure and I really feel that it works the triceps nicely. It should be done with a fairly moderate weight so that you don't place too much stress on the neck or elbows. Keep your elbow tight and in and lower the dumbbells down towards the back of the head and on the way up try to get a full contraction. I always see morons in the gym using a heavy weight and rocking their bodies and pressing the dumbbell with every stabilizer muscle possible. Then they ask me why their tri's don't grow. I am going so heavy and yet it seems to be stagnant. I just laugh and say well maybe you're doing something wrong; knowing that the only thing they are doing wrong is substituting heavy weight for form, a big NO NO. Take a dumbbell in one hand and hold it extended overhead while sitting on a bench. Keeping your elbow stationary and close to your head, lower the dumbbell down behind your head as far as you can (usually creating a 90 degree angle). Once you feel a stretch in the triceps begin to press the weight back up to the starting position. Make sure that this exercise is done as strictly as possible. Once you finish your set, then repeat the movement with the other arm. This exercise can also be done standing up by balancing yourself on to something with your free hand. I always do this exercise while facing a mirror so that way I can ensure proper form.

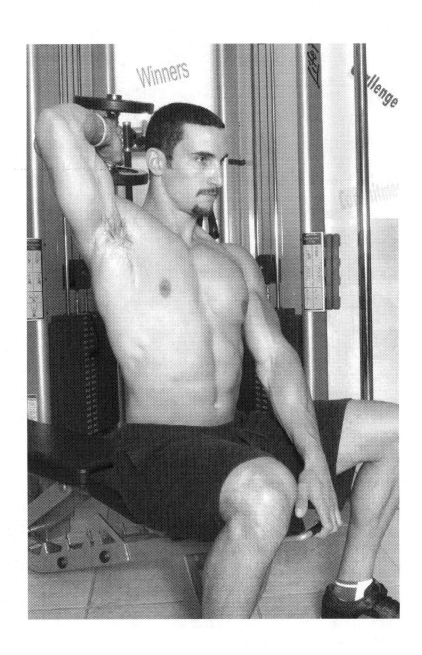

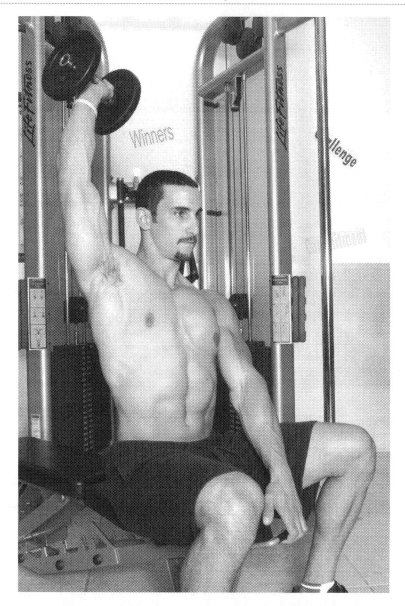

Before we move on I would just like to leave off with a side note regarding the triceps. I can't stress how important form is on the arms and how taking too much rest in between sets can be harmful to seeing results. I notice that when I am at a gym, the majority of people are waiting patiently for a machine, barbell, dumbbells or a cable unit and allowing them to cool down and rest. The triceps are a small muscle group and can rest once you pound the hell out of them. This is a common mistake I notice – most people will only wait for a cable unit to attach a piece of equipment and work their sets on. Well if that's the case then here is a bit of information – you can attach any cable attachments on any unit or machine that has a pulley and guess what, a lat machine has a pulley for you to use. This is perfect for you so that you don't wait patiently while the muscle cools down and you are now beginning to use a very important tool needed for weight training – IMPROVISATION. Work with what you have at the present moment rather than waiting and guessing how long some bum will be holding up a certain machine.

Part III – WRIST TAKER – working out your forearms and wrists

Not too many realize that forearms are a vital key to overall strength. How many times have you lifted a weight of some sort and complained that your wrists hurt? I am sure that the answer is quite a few times. The forearms get worked on almost all the time but not in an isolated manner. We use these muscles in almost every day activities besides working out and so why not make them just as strong as all the other muscles. I notice that not too many people work out their forearms a lot for a few reasons: (1) they do not know what exercises to perform (2) their excuse for not working out forearms is why do I need them (3) a common myth, they assume since they are working out their biceps it automatically works out the forearms and makes them stronger and (4) the exercises are boring and hurt my hands and fingers. The fact that number 3 has a slight truth to it makes it a bit more interesting. Like I mentioned before, whenever you work out any bodypart, especially the biceps, you are indirectly working the forearms. However, as I also mentioned before, every part of the body needs direct tension and a great amount of isolation to actually further develop them. From my experiences I have learned that once I started working out my forearms and wrists, I developed a great amount of strength in many chest and shoulder exercises. My dumbbell presses for both these bodyparts increased tremendously and I also took note that my forearms had gotten bigger and lumpier. I mean after all, think about where all the weight rests when you carry something. Exactly, on the forearms. In addition, I contribute working out forearms to developing better finger dexterity and a much better GRIP on things. So to sum things up, the exercises I recommend are:

Reverse Curls with a barbell, dumbbell or e-z curl bar. You can also use a cable machine with either an e-z bar attachment, a straight bar attachment or a single-grip handle attachment. Make sure your elbows are glued to your sides like any other arm exercise. Stand with your feet shoulder-width apart and grab a barbell with an overhand grip and hold it down in front of you at arm's length. Begin to curl the weight out and up to about almost even to your chin. Then lower the weight through a controlled motion and repeat. The reverse grip of this exercise makes the top of the forearm work extremely hard and definitely strengthens it. This exercise can also be performed on a preacher bench with a barbell, e-z bar or even a straight bar cable attachment.

Barbell

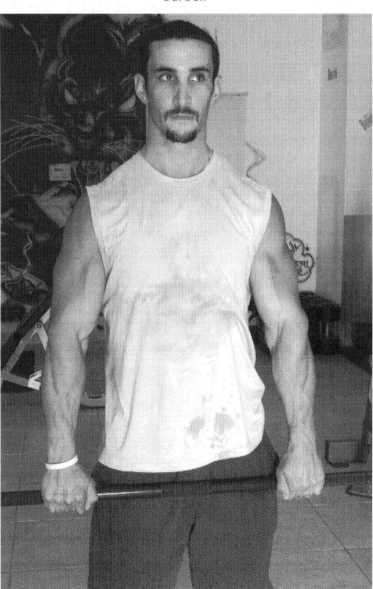

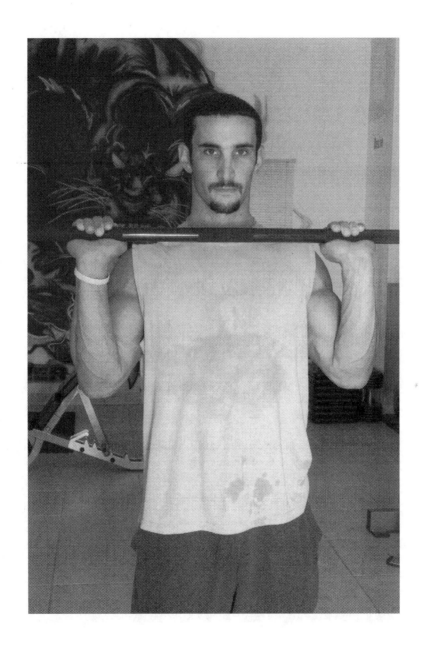

Dumbbells

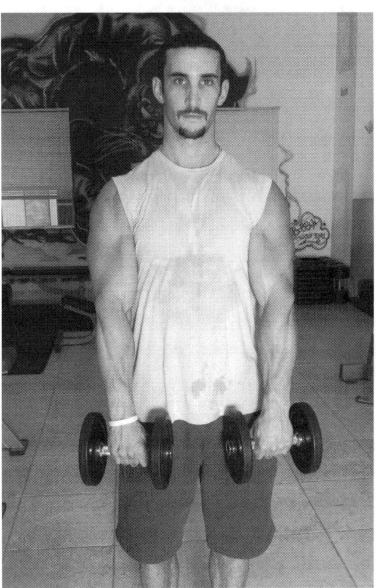

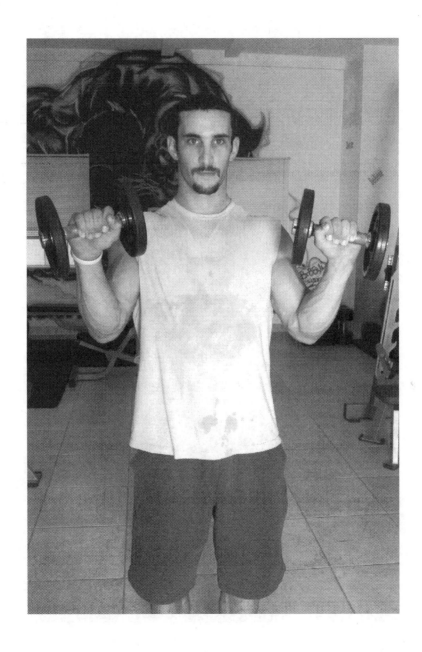

Reverse E-Z Bar Cable Curls

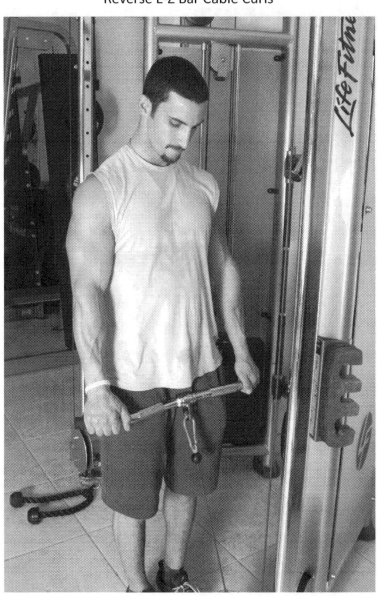

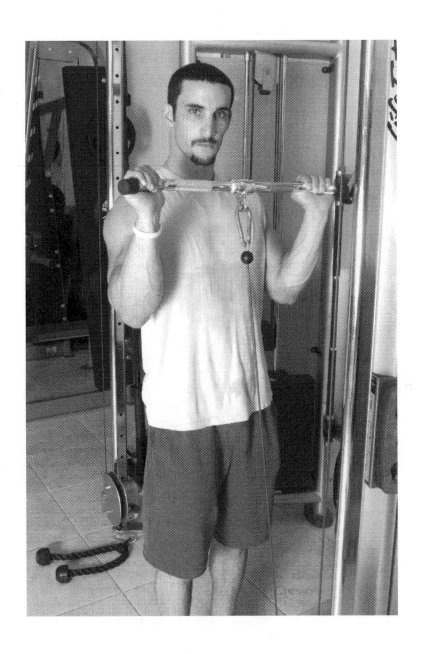

Reverse Curls using a single grip handle

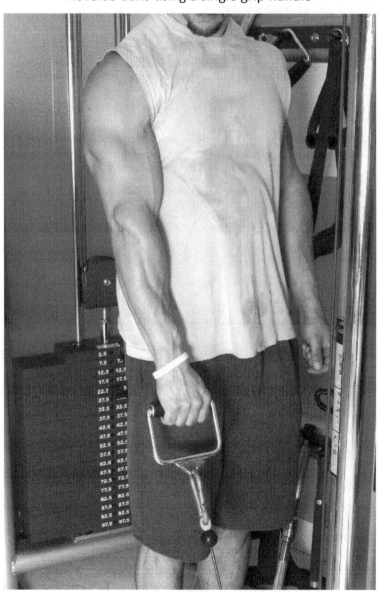

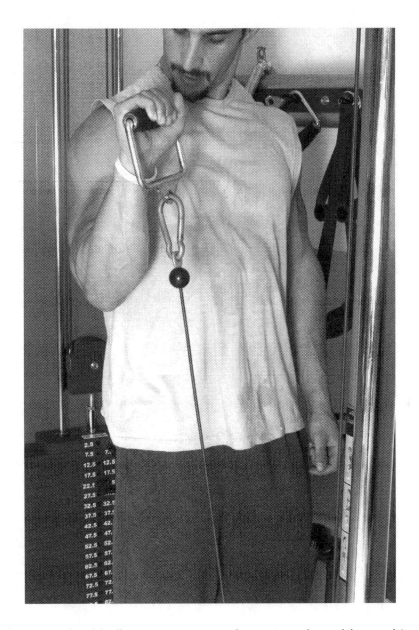

Hammer Curls using dumbbells or a rope attachment to the cable machine (previously mentioned)

Dumbbell Wrist Curls - hold the dumbbells by the side of your thighs, palms facing in and begin to curl the dumbbell. Do not bend your elbows or use any other body part.

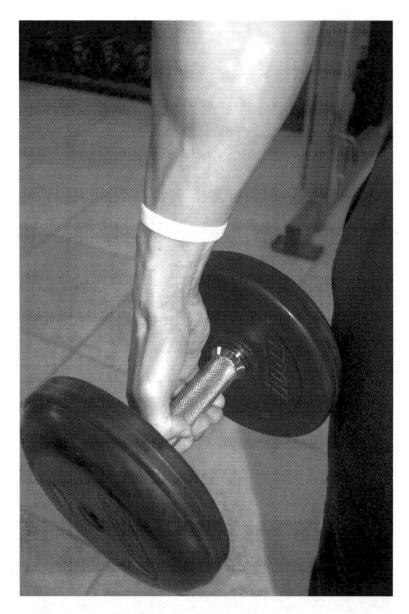

Allow the dumbbell roll down to your fingertips for maximum results. This will really build up the forearms and lead to overall finger dexterity.

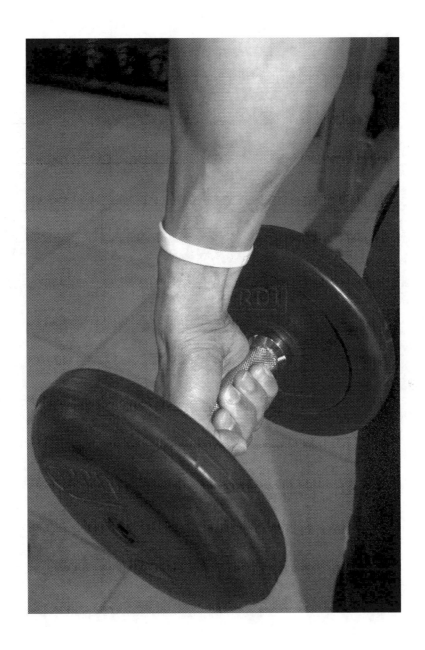

Barbell Wrist Curls (to the front and behind the back) – if you are doing this exercise behind-the-back just grab the barbell and hold it down at arm's length behind you. Your hand positioning should be about shoulder width apart with your palms facing toward the rear. Make sure your arms are steady and open your fingers and let the bar roll down out of your palms. Close your fingers and begin to roll the bar back up into your hands. Make sure to lift the bar back up as far as possible while flexing your forearms throughout the movement.

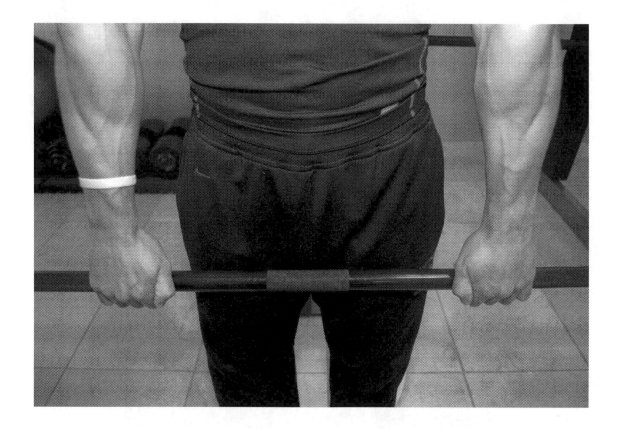

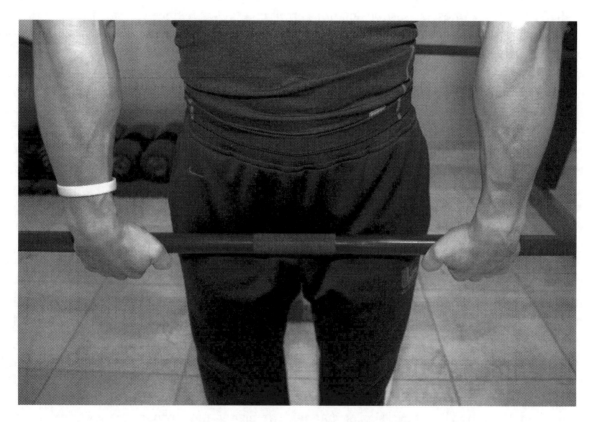

Be sure to roll the bar up as far as you possibly can. This
will really stress the forearm muscles.

Chapter 7
NO LEGGIN AROUND (Working Your Legs)

Your leg and hamstring muscles are home to the largest muscle group you have in your body. They are the muscles responsible for carrying you everywhere you go. They need to be properly trained and are just as important as every other muscle we spoke about. So we all know that the basic function of the thighs or quadriceps is to extend and straighten the leg. In addition to the quadriceps you also have the hamstrings muscle and its basic function is to curl the leg back. Below your legs you have your two calf muscles which are known as the **gastrocnemius** and the **soleus** (Later to be explained). Now I know I said that in no way will this book be filled with technical terms and words, but I think the exception for that is when talking about legs. The quadriceps consists of four muscles that make up the front of the thighs. These four heads are known as: rectus femoris, vastus lateralis, vastus medialis and vastus intermedius. Together, these four large muscles serve one purpose and one purpose only: to straighten your leg from your knee. There is no other muscle in the body that we use constantly than the legs. Something basic as walking involves a certain amount of leg effort and demand.

Like so many others in the gym, I always had a tendency to train my upper body more intense than my legs. I would look for every excuse as to why I did not want to train legs. Since the demands of leg training is so strenuous and involves pain, I, along with many others, lagged behind and never even displayed any effort. We men are so egoistic that we worry way too much on how our upper body looks and how much bigger we can get. I wish I knew then what I know now for I can assure you that my physique would have been a whole lot different. Your legs are like tree trunks; the more weight of the trunk, the more the tree can grow and branch out. Your body acts in a similar manner. The bigger and stronger the legs, the more weight it can carry on top. The minute I figured this out my legs began to take major change and my body began to grow. To think all this time my body was just waiting to grow but had no way of supporting its self on my weak and small foundation – my legs. Like any other muscle in the body, you must use correct technique for maximum results. Always pay close attention to how the exercise is performed and develop a good sense of knowledge as to what constitutes proper from. If you don't do what is told then your efforts will be wasted and your potential will never be reached.

Since there are four huge muscles that make up the quadriceps I choose certain exercises that trigger each head separately. Now if you're just looking to work out legs to become stronger, quicker, proportionate or just to increase your testosterone levels then these exercises should work. However, for those looking to become freaks of nature walking on two huge and really defined set of wheels (legs) then I will also list a few key exercises for developing them.

Part I – basic exercises for the thighs/quadriceps/quads/legs/wheels

Squats – the best exercise for overall leg development. This exercise strengthens your quadriceps, hamstrings and butt. It is a common exercise but also the most common for injuries and mistakes. If you have any type of lower back, hip injury or knee problems then try to work with a trainer to make sure that your form is 100% correct. I will list a few common mistakes that you need to avoid:

- Do not allow your knees to go past your toes

- Try to keep your head up and your eyes fixated on an object in front of you. This will allow the movement to be done with more accuracy and control

- Do not, in any way, arch your back as you stand back up

- Always try to perform this exercise in a rhythmic pace

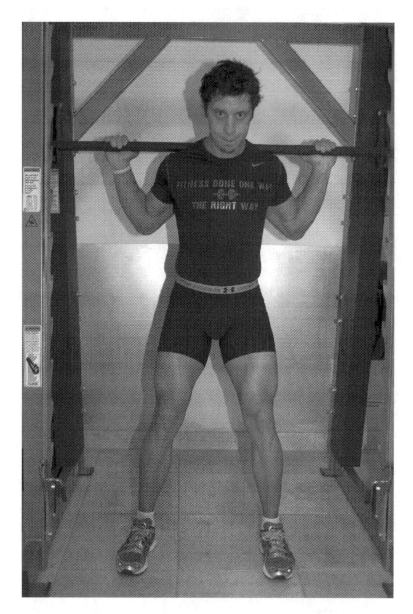

Here is the trainer performing squats on a smith machine. Notice that his back and neck are straight in effort to avoid placing stress on the lower back muscles.

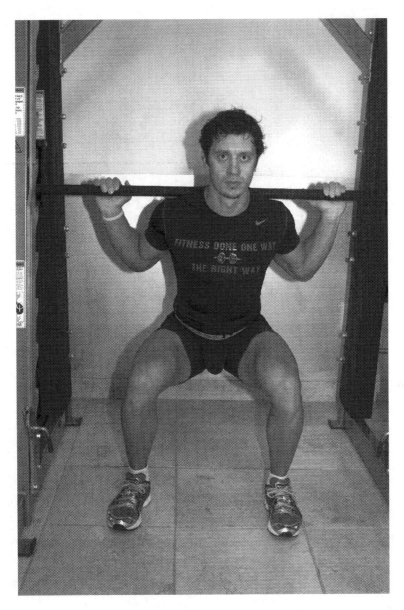

Or Barbell (either from a rack or without)

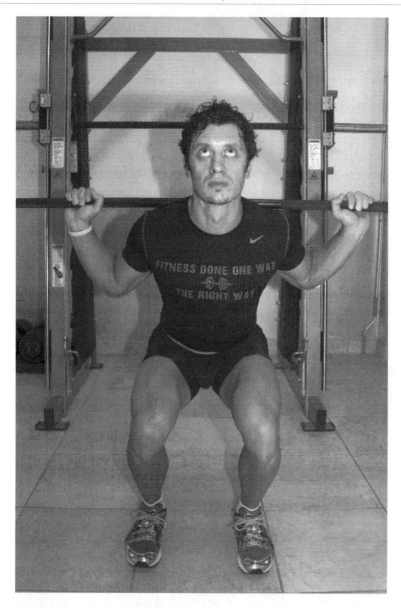

While doing a squat it is important to keep your head up at all times. While keeping your head up you are taking the pressure off of your lower back and neck and placing all the stress on the leg and butt muscles. If you are flexible and able to perform a perfect squat then make sure your knees are bent and lower yourself until your hamstrings are parallel to the floor. From this point, with all your strength push yourself up to the starting position.

In addition to the above demonstrated squats, there are three foot modifications to challenge other areas of the legs.

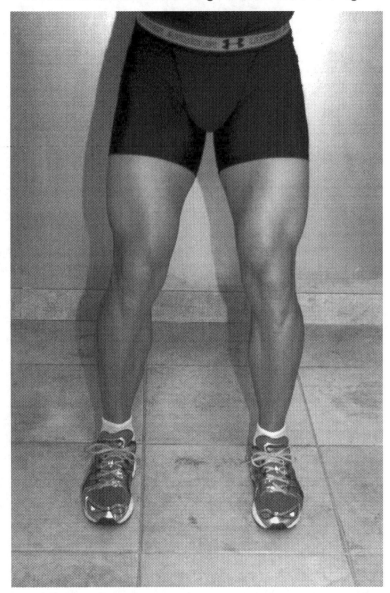

Here is an example of the common shoulder-width apart stance. It is perfect for targeting the quadriceps and the hamstrings.

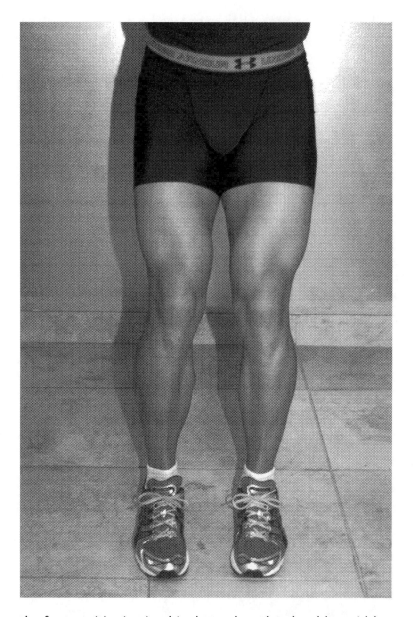

Here the foot positioning is a bit closer than the shoulder-width stance
(about 4 to 6 inches). A bit more complicated and a bit more challenging.
This stance works well for the outer thighs, glutes and quadriceps.
Not a real common position but needed to be addressed.

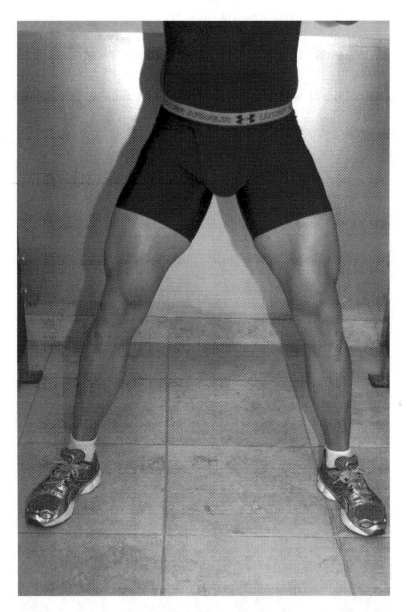

This is the most common position I see performed. It is real easy on the back and places a great deal of tension on the inner thighs, glutes and hamstrings. Very easy to squat heavy in this position.

Lunges – another great overall leg exercise. Just like squats, it strengthens your quadriceps, hamstrings and butt. Make sure you keep good balance towards the entire movement. This is a great exercise for not only legs, but for coordination, stability, balance and posture. As you get more inclined to this exercise, you can now change your options and your positioning. Before this you were doing a regular lunge keeping one leg stationary (of course bent) and bending the other. Now you can pick from four different options:

Lunges with either a weighted bar on the back of your neck or holding dumbbells at your sides.

Barbell

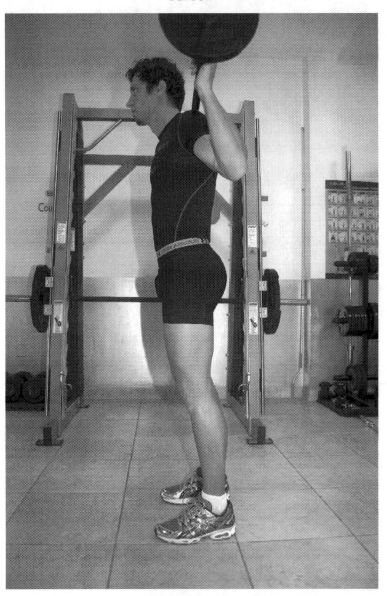

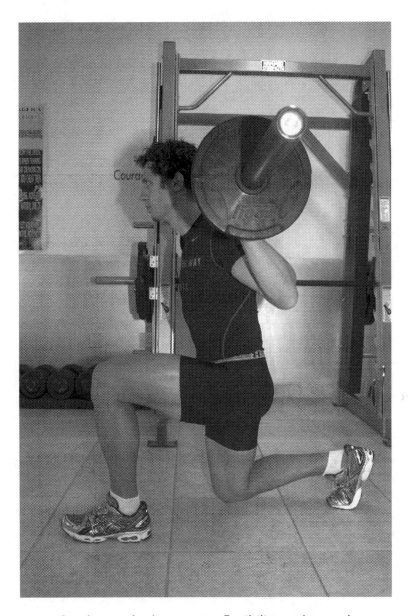

Or for those who have more flexibility and can take a
longer stride the picture below is for you.

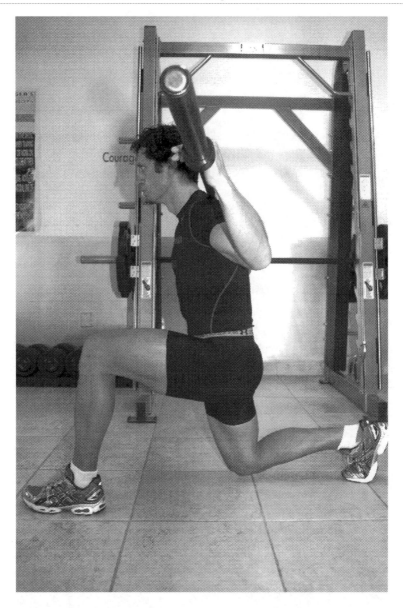

Lunges with either a smith machine or a barbell – this is a bit more serious and demands more strength and coordination. While performing this exercise you can alternate legs (hard) or keep one leg stationary. Both are effective and a real pain in the butt, literally.

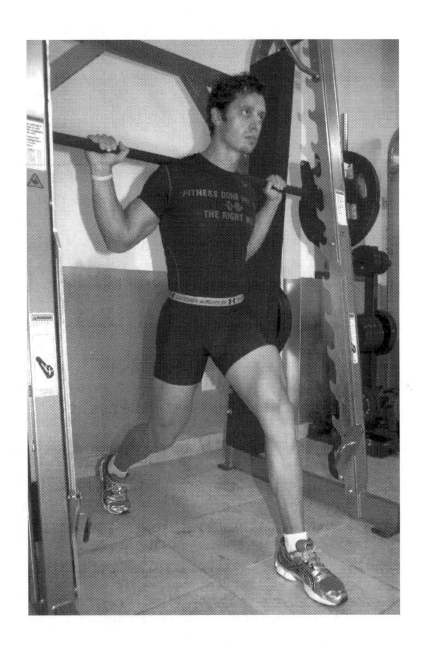

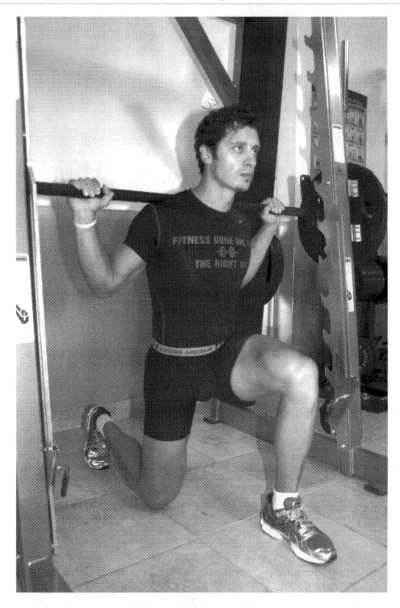

Walking lunges – you perform the basic lunge, with the exception of alternating legs and traveling forward with each repetition. Make sure you can walk at least 10 strides and maintain balance throughout the set.

Reverse lunges or backwards lunges – same motion as a regular forward lunge except you now do it backwards. Instead of stepping forward just step back. A challenging exercise because it definitely involves a great amount of coordination. You can also make it even more challenging by using a step board or a elevated platform. This changes the tension on the hamstrings and glutes. Some also refer this exercise as a Bulgarian Deadlift/Lunge.

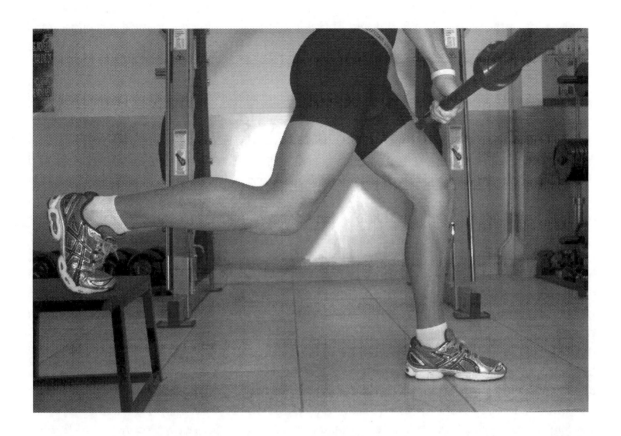

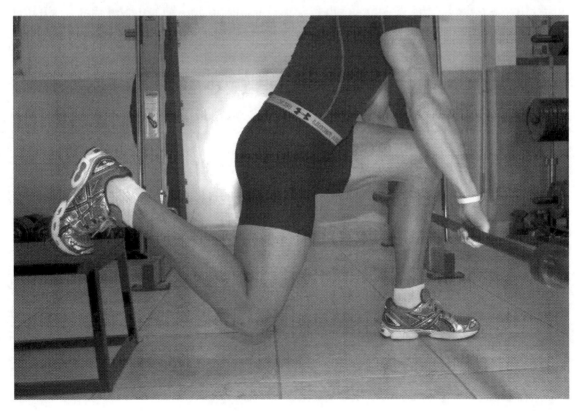

Leg Presses – if all else fails for you then this exercise should be your number 1 priority. It covers a lot of ground and develops the entire leg muscle. Many gyms have a few versions of this machine. The old fashioned version of the leg press is still in use and only looks a bit smaller. So at first glance this huge contraption doesn't scare many people away – thanks to the advancements in gym equipment. The majority of these machines are plate loaded, meaning that if you're a lazy person then walk on over to the weight stack and move the pin in and out of your desired weight on a different machine. As noted there are a few of these leg press machines you might come across. Don't freak out and get all nervous, each machine can be geared for that person. The only thing I can tell you is that the motion is the same and the emphasis of the exercise is the same – to build mass and strength on the thighs. Squats and lunges are great but have one disadvantage – put tons of pressure on your lower back. Leg presses allow you work around the pressure and even go heavy.

Leg Extensions – this is defined as more of a shaping/sculpting exercise. It is a great way to begin a session of legs since it lubricates the joints well. Also from my experiences the leg extensions were great for developing the area around my knees and extremely helpful in getting me more defined. Most of my clients over the years felt that I was only torturing them when I told them to do a set of 20 or 25 repetitions and repeat it for 3 or 4 sets. To execute this exercise correctly make sure that your butt is flat on the chair and is not lifting up after every repetition. You want this motion to be as strict and correct as possible. Once seated and secured under the padded bar, extend your legs to maximum extension. Extend your legs out till the point where your knees are locked. When I say locked, try to still keep a slight bend in the knee while extending for a maximum contraction. Once you contract at the top you can begin to lower the weight slowly to the starting position. I am sure that if you do it in the correct form your legs will begin to burn immensely.

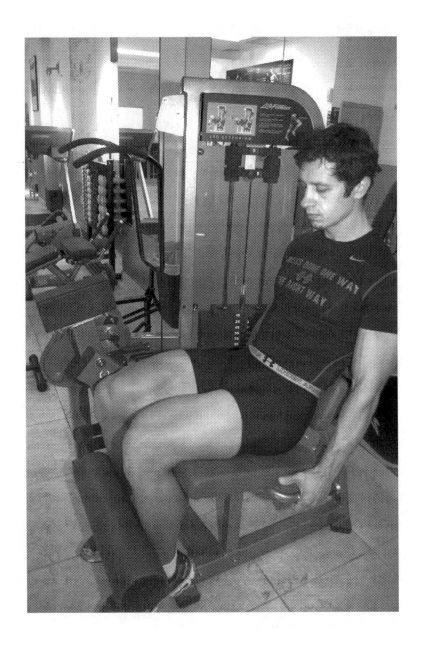

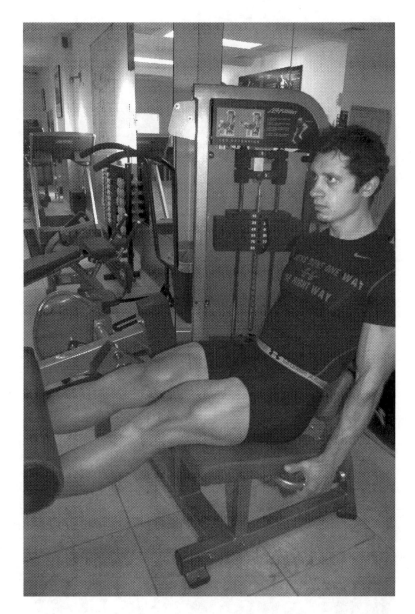

Or you can try to change your foot positioning to target other areas
(feet close together and toes pointed out and wide)

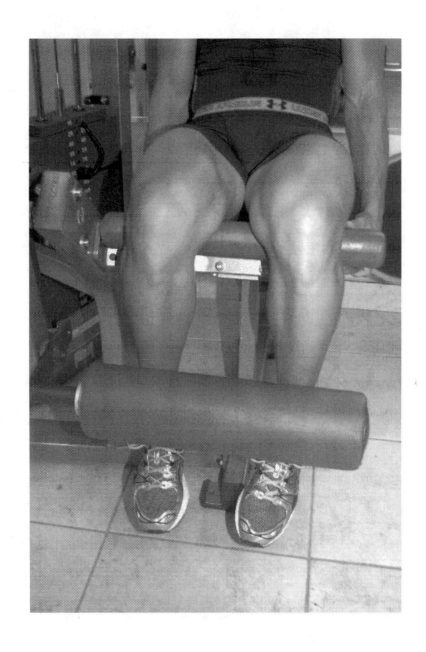

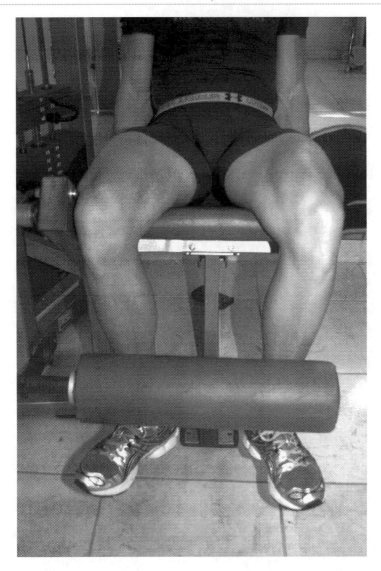

Leg Curls – the leg curl machine is a phenomenal piece of equipment for strengthening the hamstring and butt muscles. Lay face down on the machine and make sure to hook your heels on the padded bar. At this point your legs should be straight out and completely stretched. While keeping your entire body on the bench, begin to curl your legs up as far as possible (about 90 degrees) to ensure a good contraction of the hamstring muscle. Then lower the weight slowly and controlled to its starting position.

Many gyms have a few leg curl machines handy for you to use. The only difference I noticed over the years is that some are different in colors and some have a slightly different angle. However, the motion should be constant and uniform for every angle and color. That is why it is crucial for proper form and control so that you can apply it to any type of machine. In addition, many gyms have a different leg curl machine, known as a standing leg curl. I know I said that there is not that much difference in between these machines and I was right; well except for the fact that you don't lay face down on the standing leg curl. You stand against the machine and hook one leg under the padded bar and curl up. Make sure that you hold good posture and keep yourself steady while doing a repetition.

Stiff-Legged Deadlifts - the purpose of this compound exercise is to develop your hamstrings, butt and lower back. It is a challenging exercise but has excellent benefits. You can perform this exercise with either holding dumbbells in front of you or using a barbell. Take hold of the weight and begin at a standing position. You want to make sure that your legs are at least shoulder width apart and you're back is straight. Once you have a good grasp of the bar or dumbbells, keeping your knees locked, bend forward from the waist and try to touch your toes. For those who have a greater range of motion try to use either some sort of block or bench as a way to allow for a maximum extent on the bottom of the movement. Make sure your back is at all times straight and at no point should it begin to round.

Dumbbells

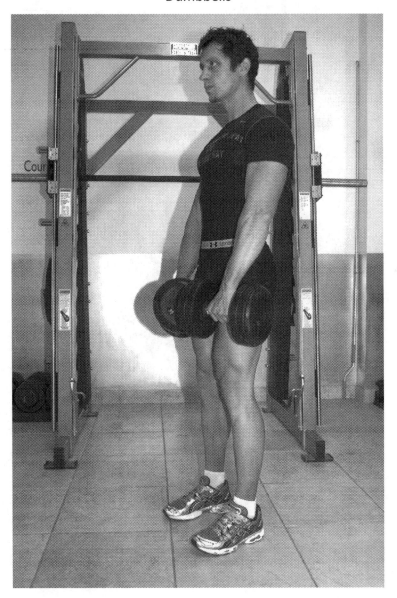

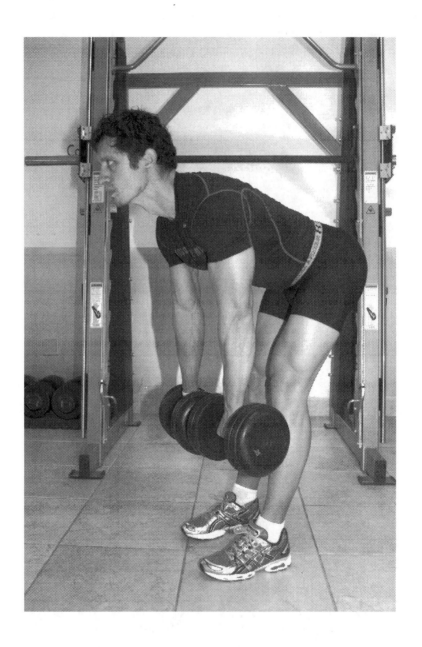

Barbell

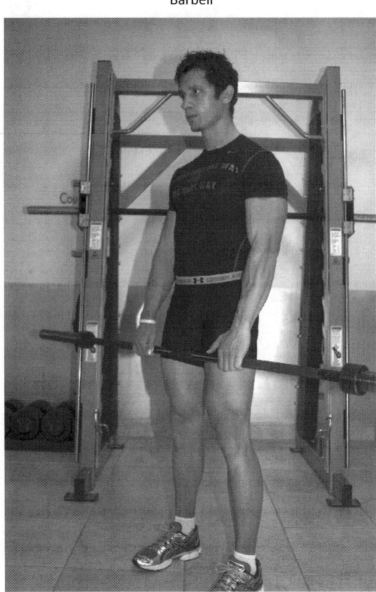

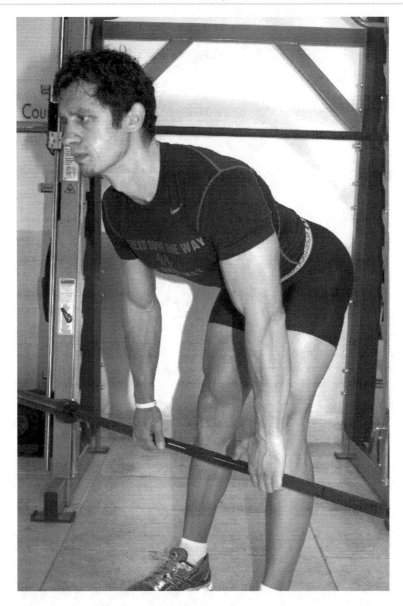

Inner/Outer Thigh Machine (hip abductors)

This is a great piece of equipment for both men and women. It does a great job strengthening the inner thigh muscles and the outer thigh muscles. It is a great machine for flexibility and prevention of injury. There are a few other exercises that can be improvised with this but I totally urge you to use these machines for maximum results. In addition, it will greatly help you squat in the long run.

Part II – Big legs – almost like 24 inch rims on a car

So now that we covered mostly all of the basic leg exercises for an average person, let's talk about leg exercises for those who want really huge legs. All of the exercises listed above are going to be used with the exception of one or two more exercises. Since the quadriceps is a large muscle group the major differences for average people trying to stay fit and healthy and bodybuilders are foot positioning and weight capacity. The difference in the way your toes are pointing is a major issue. Till now you got used to toes slightly pointed out and shoulder width apart. This is no longer the case – the best three and common positions are (1) toes pointed slightly out (2) toes pointed straight ahead (very challenging and places a great deal of pressure on the lower back) and (3) toes pointed out at a wide angle. These three positions are great in achieving that define and striated look you have been dreaming of. A good amount of variety in these positions is crucial to achieving overall development of the thigh muscle. I learned this stuff only after the first time I came across the bible of bodybuilding and that is *THE NEW ENCYCLOPEDIA OF MODERN BODYBUILDING BY ARNOLD SCHWARZENEGGER.* This book is a classic and everyone should own it. The information contained in this book is so vast and informative that no other book will ever come close to. I was blown away with endless pages of information and images. Arnold is and will always be a true icon in the sense of fitness, bodybuilding, acting, writer, and politician. As a matter of fact, every time I look at his book (almost daily) I get such a rush and an urge to work out legs. I do think that my book is extremely informative and motivational as well.

Another great exercise for developing the thigh muscle is the hack squat machine. Similar to a squat, this exercise is great for developing the lower area of the thigh; the area by the knee. Your back goes against a pad and your shoulders locked under the padded bars. Once you're situated and your toe position is determined, press downwards bending your legs and try to make your hamstrings parallel to the floor or to the platform of the machine. Make sure that your back is on the pad at all times while going up and down on this machine. The second great exercise for mass that not too many people do are front squats. So are you a bit nervous from this exercise? I was. I mean you are doing a squat except for the fact that the bar is now being carried on your front deltoids with your arms grasping the bar to control it. This is a challenging exercise and might take some use getting to. I mean just think about it, you are placing all the weight on your front thighs and boy do you feel it. Be sure to have your toes pointed slightly out and your back straight to achieve proper form. The third exercise great for developing mass is the leg press. Now we mentioned this exercise before except now we know that foot positioning and weight is the ultimate goal for mass. Don't be afraid to load up the bar with weight and have your toes either pointed out or just pointed straight ahead and close together. This is definitely a great way to build mass around the outside and inside sweep of the quadriceps. So now that we got all the exercises and foot positions out the way we can discuss the calves.

Example of Front Squats

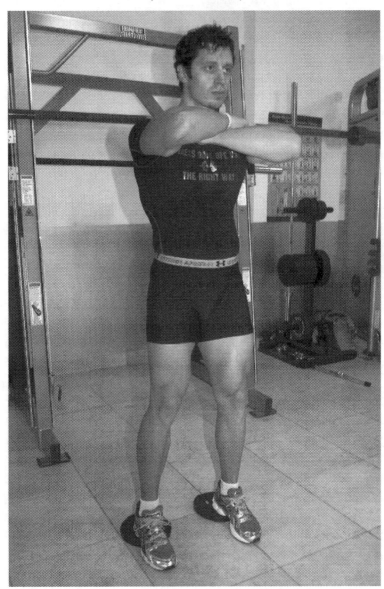

Make sure that the bar is situated comfortably on your deltoids.

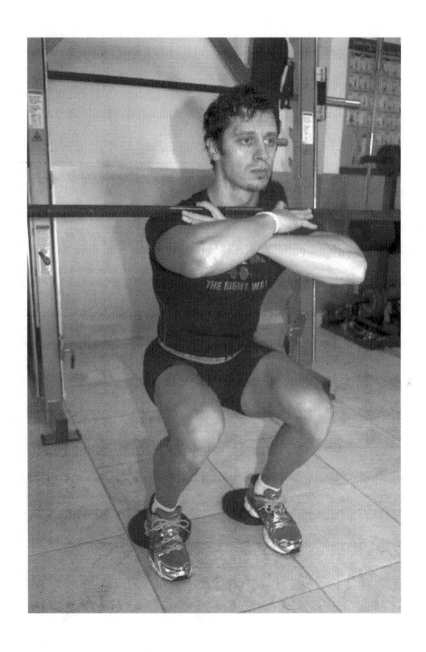

Part III – Grow Calves Grow – training that stagnant muscle we call Calves

The calves, one of the hardest muscles to develop, have become real popular over the years. I mean you now begin to see calf muscles in all shapes and sizes. For these professional bodybuilders calf development is a major issue and is looked at thoroughly when being judged. We understand that they are considered the hardest muscle group in the body to develop but can respond effectively to training like any other muscle. A great amount of technique, exercises, weight and angles need to be at the forefront for great calf development. It is sad to say that without good calves your physique cannot be complete. Yes I have heard that they are a stagnant muscle group or that I do almost everything and still not see them grow and even at times I hear that they don't grow because of my genes. Of course all these are excuses I believed till recently. I started to believe that you get only good calves if you either got implants or just injected your calves with some powerful anabolics. I was not ready to do that nor was I ready to spend 30 to 45 minutes of heavy calf training. Such a small bodypart does not need that much work. Boy was I wrong. It's the opposite – the calves need to be treated like any other body part. They need to be put through constant work and hit from every angle. You must remember that since they are a small muscle group they tend to recuperate much quicker than other body parts. Therefore, you can even train them every other day if you desired. So we understand that the calves are tough and can stand a lot of heavy weight and work, so you must use different machines, angles and shock this hard-to-grow muscle. Until I trained my calves the right way, the way Arnold Schwarzenegger describes, I had trouble getting my calves as big and ripped as I wanted them. Once I learned certain words like high-intensity, shocking principle, partial reps, staggered sets and so many others I began to notice immediate changes. If you are willing to pay the price and endure serious hours of proper training for calves then you will see results and even have some people admire both your hard work ethics and your calf development.

So before I list a few calf exercises lets recap: it is very important to get a full range of motion, meaning you get a full stretch at the bottom and then up on your toes for a full contraction. This stays the same for every different exercise and every different toe positioning. Make sure to use heavy weight that is manageable and attempt to maintain proper form and strict contractions throughout every repetition and every set. In addition to these two rules, make sure you work your calves at least three times a week with a solid program. Do not rush through your calf workout and do a few sets as a means to complete your workout. If you are not ready to set aside time for calves then don't even bother with a few sets because it's useless.

Calf Exercises

Standing Calf Raises – a great exercise to develop the overall mass and shape of the calves. Many gyms have a few of these machines and the weight stack on them is pretty heavy. I've seen the weight go up to 400 pounds in one gym. You start off with your feet on the block/bar/platform with your shoulders under the pads and standing upright. Once you are secured and your foot position is determined you lower your heels as far down as possible while keeping your knees slightly bent throughout the movement. Once your heels are totally stretched you begin to come up on your toes as far as possible maximizing a full contraction at the top of the movement. Remember, you can perform this exercise and many others either in the toes-in position, the toes-out position or toes-straight position.

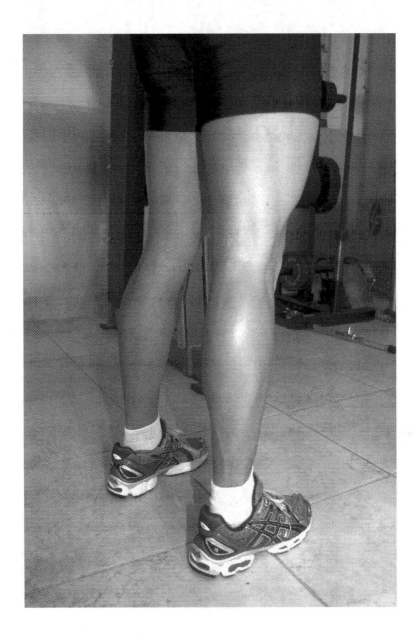

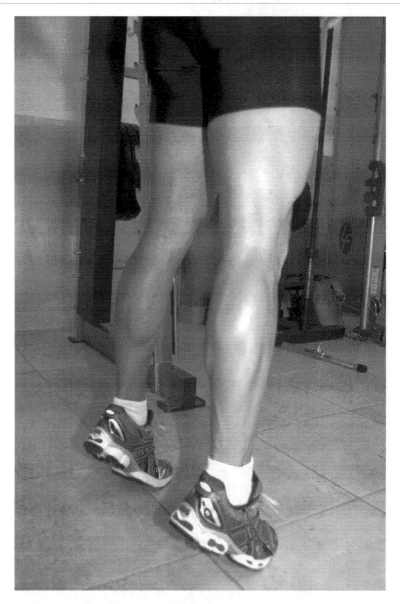

Seated Calf Raises – another calf machine favorite. Sit on the machine with your knees under a pad or crossbar and begin to lower your heels to the ground and then back up to full contraction. Make sure your posture is straight and do not rock back and forth throughout the movement.

Calf Raises on a Leg Press Machine – this allows you to go super heavy since the safety bars are in place in case your toes slip. While doing this exercise make sure you are able to get a full stretch of your muscle while lowering your heels. Once you feel that stretch begin to press upwards with your toes as far as possible.

These are the three most commonly used machines you will find in a gym or fitness center. You can get a great workout if you use these three exercises with high intensity, good weight and a great variety in toe positioning.

Chapter 8
ABSolutely Amazing – Working Your Abdominals

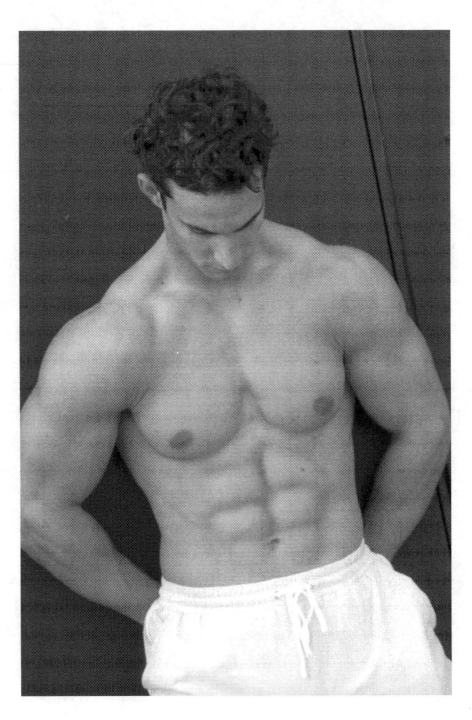

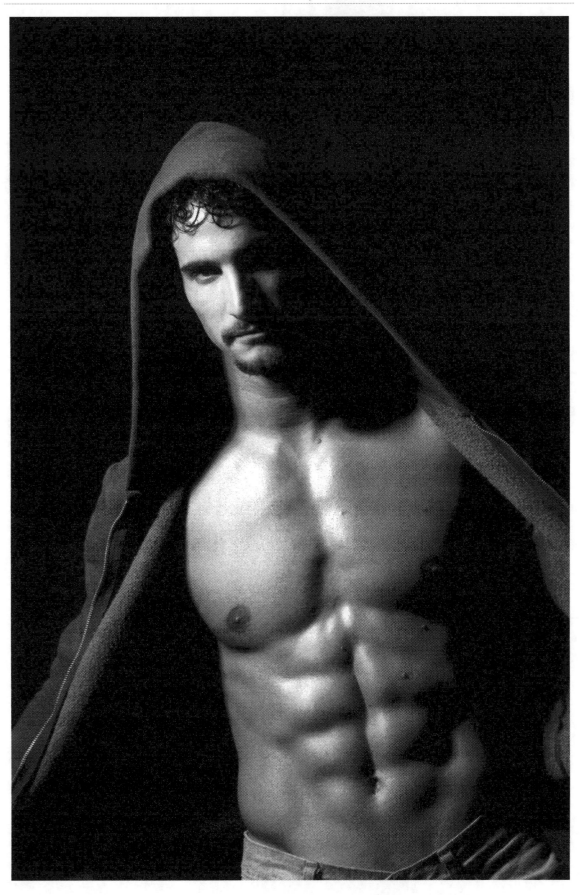

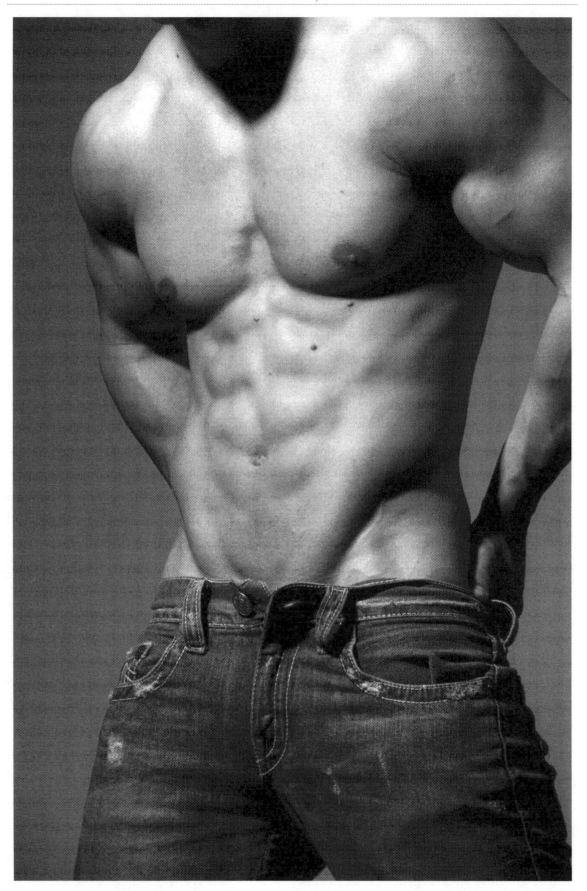

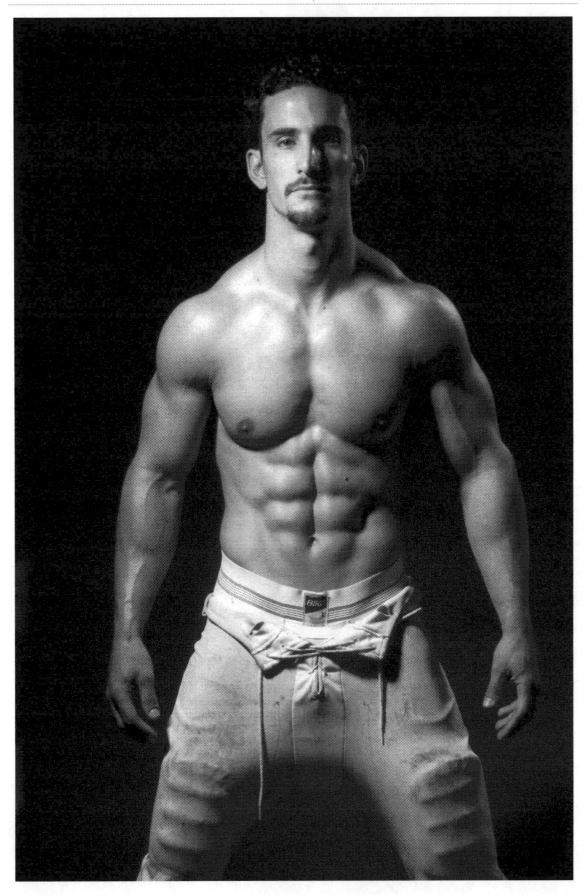

For those who don't know, your abdominal region is the most visible part of the body. It is the center of attention. It is the ultimate goal for one to develop a six pack, and I don't mean a six pack of beer. The abdominal region is a bit complex and has many myths and fabrications regarding it. It is because of this that all those fancy television ads displaying their gizmos bank roll every year. Fancy slogans and fit models will always do the trick. I mean as your eating that ice cream or bag of chips you think to yourself wow, I can be eating these foods while performing a few sets on these gizmos. I mean how dumb can you be? These items are directly geared for those lazy people who look for the easy way out and want to cut corners. There are at least twenty gadgets that I came across when writing this book and all were absolutely useless, retarded and a waste of money. AbTrainer, AbRoller, AbRocket and so many others are just a few of the names I came across. I just can't understand how people get so sucked in and just throw money away to all those infomercials that simply brainwash the individual. Oh well, welcome to the wonderful world of capitalism. No one said it has to be true and no one definitely said that it has to be effective. All it takes is a patent, some money and a few egoistic models and you got yourself a great selling item.

The abdominals consist of four muscles – the *Rectus Abdominis, the External Obliques, the Internal Obliques, and the Intercostals.* However, all people in every household and gym in America refers to these muscles as the ABS. The importance of strong abdominals is sometimes over looked. They are absolutely essential to almost every sport and every movement and play a crucial role for overall appearance. Just remember that your abdominals support your spine in all movements. Over the years your abdominal region has been linked to core training and functional training. These type of workouts help tighten both your abdominals and lower back. They help in getting you that strength you need to have good posture and a real strong mid-section. In other words, your lower back and your abs work hand-in-hand. A strong mid-section will ensure a strong lower back and vice versa. This is because since the abdominals and obliques support your spine they also dictate your posture. If you tend to lean forward or sag forward then chances are you're going to throw your lower back off kilter. Then at this point you begin to realize that you're in desperate need of core training placing more importance to the abdominals. In addition to all that was mentioned, you will now begin to stand up straight with confidence and may even gain a six pack (if you work harder). I can guarantee you that once you achieve this six pack the babes will begin to go wild. Wow becomes a common word you begin to hear. I still have girls walk over to me and ask me if they can use my stomach as a wash board. I love that feeling but only in the sense of accomplishment and not a conceited thing. It takes a real amount of dedication; commitment and passion to achieve a perfect physique so why not reap the benefits.

To truly understand the dynamics of effective abdominal training, you need to differentiate the truth from the myths. Don't go by what you heard on TV or what someone told you. I will try to go over a few of these myths while at the same time stating some truths and facts.

Myth #1: Doing abdominal exercises will get rid of my fat?

Truth: Any abdominal exercise you do will not rid get of all your fat as some infomercials might suggest. Losing body fat in this area requires much more than abdominal crunches.

It requires proper nutrition, proper supplementation and a well designed exercise program. You can only really strengthen and tone your abs but in no way will you become lean and slender. The blubber or flab around your waist takes much more time and effort to eliminate than a credit card consolidator.

Myth #2: My friend told me that if I do a few hundred crunches a day I can expect that six pack in no time.

Truth: The truth is that your friend is a telling a lie and has no clue when it comes to abdominal training. If you invest a few minutes a day doing useless crunches and ab exercises then chances are you will never get the results you desired. You must treat your abs like any other muscle group – they will only respond best to hard work and proper exercises. After all I am sure that the crunches you were doing were either done incorrectly or way too easy for you. Hence, this book is perfect for you since it will give you a good variety of exercises and how to properly execute them.

Myth #3: If I design a good program and do abs every day I will see results.

Truth: This has two answers – (1) since the abdominals are like any other muscle group they require adequate rest and recuperation after an intense workout. If you do them daily then chances are you will over train them and not see immediate results and (2) depending on the individual and his/her eating regiment doing abs daily can lead to seeing some results. This is almost like a phenomenon and worked in my case for the first few years. I would blast my abs daily with different angles and exercises and was able to get serious results. However, as the years went by I noticed that I needed a break every other day or so to maintain my eight-pack. Yes I have an eight-pack. Sometimes the correct answer is "less is always more."

Myth #4: If I use some type of ab machine or gadget I will maximize my results.

Truth: If you use a gadget or even a machine specifically designed for your abdominals you might be doing more good to your back then to your abs. These machines and gadgets usually take the stress off your abs and place it either on your lower back or hips. Not really what you want and nowhere near as effective as your traditional workouts on the floor or a mat.

Myth #5: Sit-ups' are better for results than crunches.

Truth: Nothing works better, in my opinion, then a proper crunch. With the motion of a sit-up you involve the lower back and hip muscles. Remember, you want all the stress of the contraction to target the abdominals and abdominals only.

Myth #6: If I do aerobic classes and Zumba I can get those washboard abs I have been dreaming of.

Truth: Zumba, a recent fitness revolution has people all over the world in a craze. Since it blends both dance moves and body defining movements it has become a great way to get that excitement you need in your workouts. I watch these Zumba infomercials almost every

Sunday morning and still not a true believer to gaining results. The music is hot and the dancing is wild but I am old school and believe that you need specific training for every area of your body. No one ever said that fitness is fun and I definitely don't think that dancing will get me results. However, in this day and age anything is possible and I am not knocking Zumba and its founder, rather I am sticking to my guns and being more of a realist. Your abdominals need constant contractions and workouts that I believe you can only get in a gym setting. In addition, the models they have on these Zumba commercials are just absolutely perfect. I mean real defined and a chiseled mid-section and I am sorry to say that not everyone has that body and probably won't get that body doing Zumba. Every individual is different and dynamic in their own ways. Some need more Core training, functional training or even some sort of rehabilitation so how can Zumba cater to all these people. The gym is the best answer and I know why – the equipment that you find in a gym is usually from big companies such as Life Fitness, Hammer Strength, Icarian, Cybex and a few others. These huge companies have millions and invest millions in designing equipment suitable for almost every body type, weight, height and needs so that you can get a solid workout. If these pieces of equipment did not work so well and only took up space then these companies would not be around anymore and we all would be ordering these Zumba DVD's and dancing to real good Latin music. I have taken my share of aerobic classes, sculpting classes and other such classes and the only thing I noticed was that my endurance was not as good as I thought. I did not see a six-pack after a week nor did I begin to take notice in my arms and back becoming defined. I mean these classes are a great way to strengthen your heart. Cardiovascular exercises can be great and can be performed outside the gym as well. So go ahead and make that heart strong but eventually we all need a gym to work out in and get results.

Now up to this point I have mentioned many exercises along with proper form but the basic crunch is one of the most often incorrectly performed exercise. Everyone complains of neck problems, lower back problems and occasional breathing issues. Below I will list a few mistakes to avoid when training your abdominals.

- Avoid putting stress on your neck; in other words only lift from your abs and keep your eyes fixated on an object up in the sky. Both your head and neck should not be involved in the exercise.

- Try to breathe while doing crunches. Holding your breathe will do you no justice and will definitely fatigue you quickly. I always recommend to my clients that they keep their mouths a drop open so that oxygen can come in and go out. Since crunches is a basic exercise and the starting point to other exercises you should really inhale and exhale in a rhythmic pace. Maybe count your repetitions out loud so that you are indirectly allowing yourself to breathe. I can assure you that once you learn how to breathe properly you will be much better off and able to sustain for a longer time.

- For those who feel more comfortable interlocking their fingers and placing their hands behind their necks, don't move your elbows. If you begin to move your elbows while performing a crunch then you directly place a great amount of stress on the neck. This stress can be painful and can lead you in the direction of never attempting crunches again. Leave your elbows right where they are (flared out) and only crunch using your abdominals and oblique's. I cannot stress how important this piece of information is – I have heard so many people complain and tell me that they feel more pain in their necks then their abs. Definitely not a good sign when your client pre-fatigues his/her neck before even feeling a slight burn or pain in their abdominals.

- Always do a full crunch – crunches are really just a short movement but some people forget that it actually involves lifting your shoulder blades and curling forward. Even if it's a short/small motion your neck and back should not be the only thing lifting and moving. Do the repetition correctly and maintain that form throughout.

- Always remember that ab exercises require slow, controlled and proper form. You need to maximize a full range of motion and strive for full or peak contractions.

Part I – Basic Exercises – most commonly performed exercises

Crunches – the most basic form of exercise and yet the one hardest to do. Most people have a real tough time learning how to isolate one section of the abdominal region and I guess end up getting frustrated. Crunches can be performed on the floor, on a bench or even on an old school roman chair machine. They are all effective and all work the absolute same way. Lie on your back with your knees slightly bent and feet flat on the mat or floor. Place your hands behind your neck but do not interlock your fingers or you can place your hands crossed against your chest. Once you have done this begin to lift your shoulders and neck off the mat and pull your abdominals in. A normal crunch is a short repetition so make sure you keep your chin high and try to alleviate all the pressure off your neck and onto the abdominals. While pulling your abs in make sure to get a good contraction and then easily return to starting position. A word of advice, don't let your shoulders hit the mat or floor so that way you are keeping the abs fully tensed and tight. I promise you will feel a burn much quicker this way then you would if you lowered your shoulders all the way down.

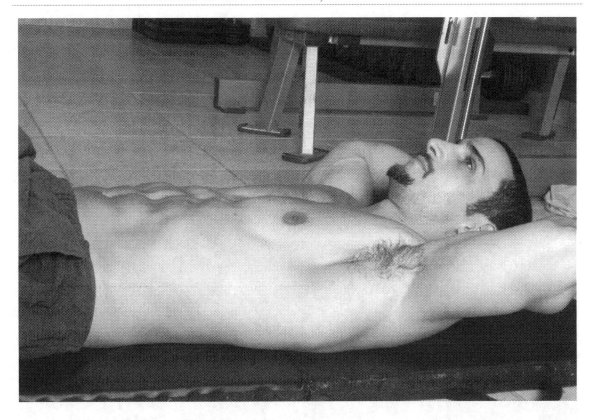

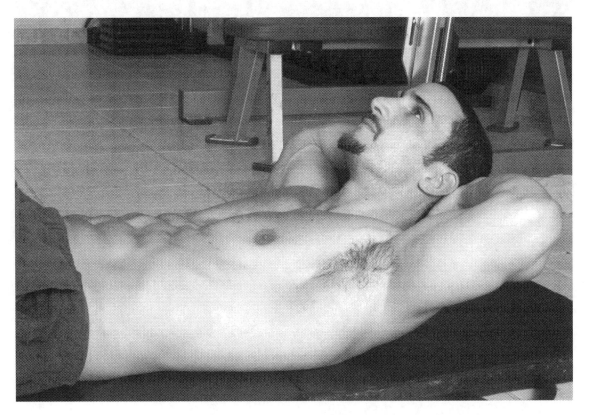

Notice that my neck is completely relaxed and the pressure
and stress is placed on my abdominals

Crunches can also be performed in different versions. You can do the traditional crunches with your knees slightly bent or you can change the focus around and do crunches with either your legs straight up or legs bent in the middle. This will begin to work the upper and lower muscles in the abdominals. Another great form of crunches that work the obliques as well is twisting crunches. Same form and routine as your basic crunch except for the fact that you are twisting your torso so that the opposite elbow comes across towards your opposite knee (ex: left elbow into right knee).Continue to alternate in one direction and then the other throughout your full set. In addition you can do the same foot positioning with this exercise as I mentioned with the basic crunch - legs straight up with a twist and legs in the middle with a twist. Only difference is that more tension is applied once your feet come off the floor.

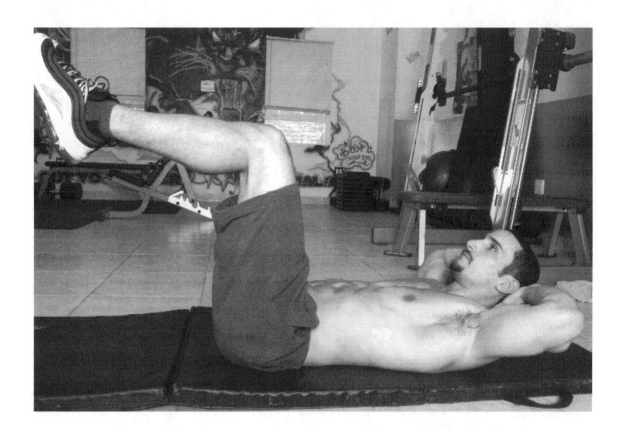

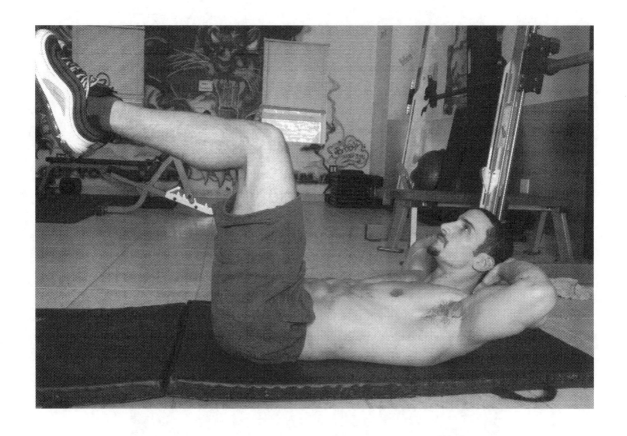

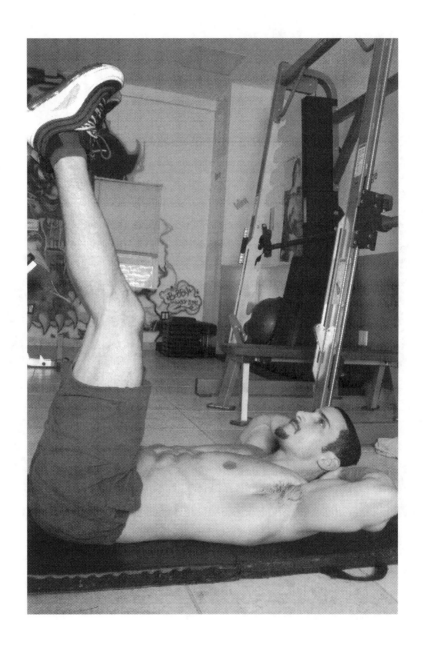

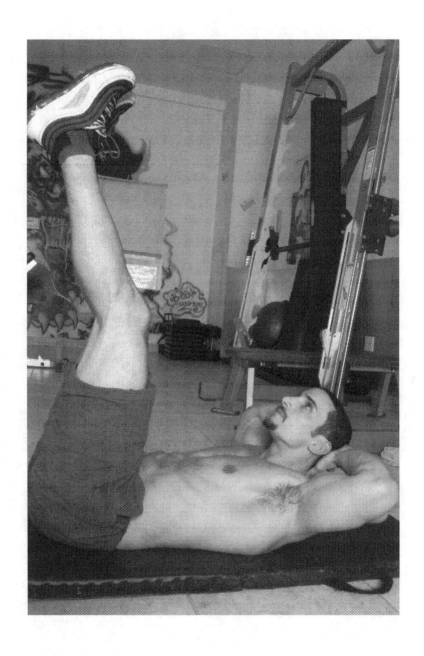

Crunches on a decline bench or Roman chair – the purpose of this exercise is to emphasis the upper region of the abs. Sit on the bench and hook your feet under the support bar and keep your arms in front of you or behind your neck. Make sure that you stomach is tucked in and lower yourself slowly and controlled then begin to raise and curl your torso forward as far as possible.

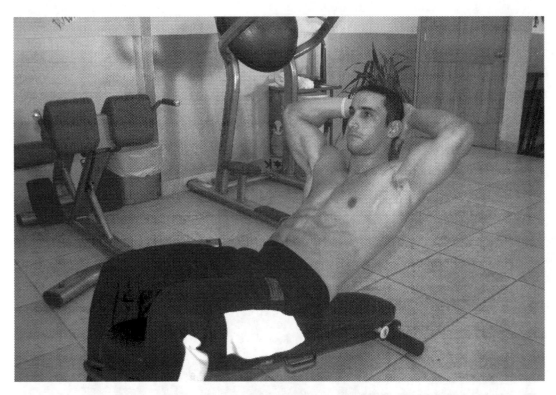

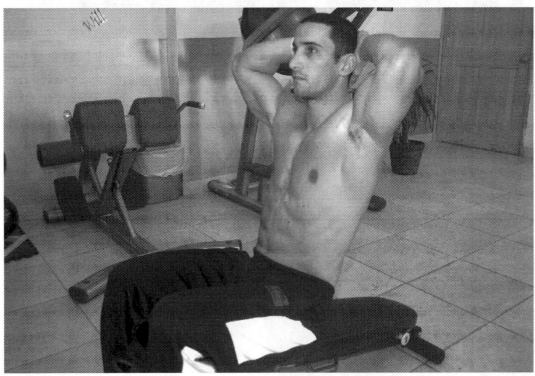

You can also do this exercise for the obliques. It is the same movement with the exception of a twist at the end/top.

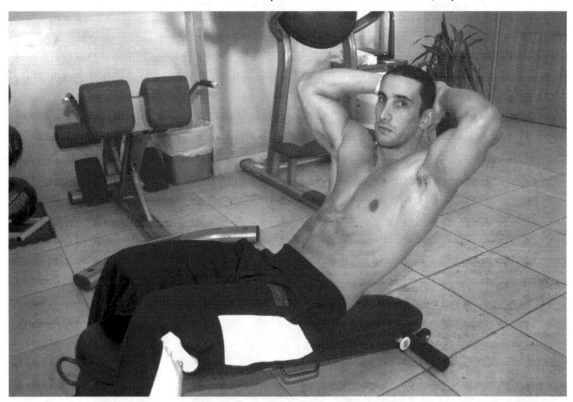

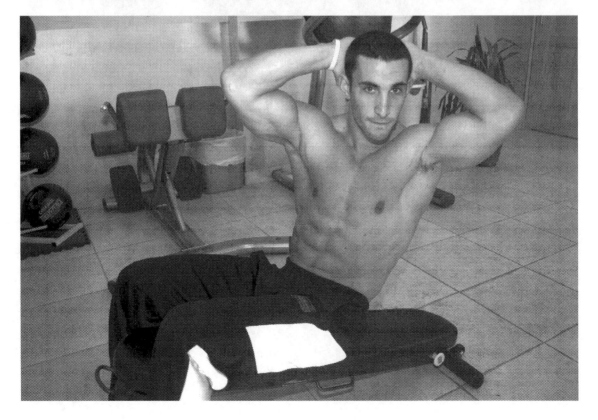

Hanging Crunches (or reverse crunches) – This exercise places a great amount of stress on the lower part of the abs. It is usually performed on a hanging bar or a pull up bar. Hold the bar in a comfortable position shoulder width apart and bring your knees up to the abdomen and really try to hold it up a second. This will definitely give you a good contraction before you lower your legs back to its starting position. Make sure your back is straight and in no means are you rocking and/or using momentum to ensure a full and proper range of motion. This can also be done with your legs straight out – which in essence adds more resistance and makes the exercise difficult.

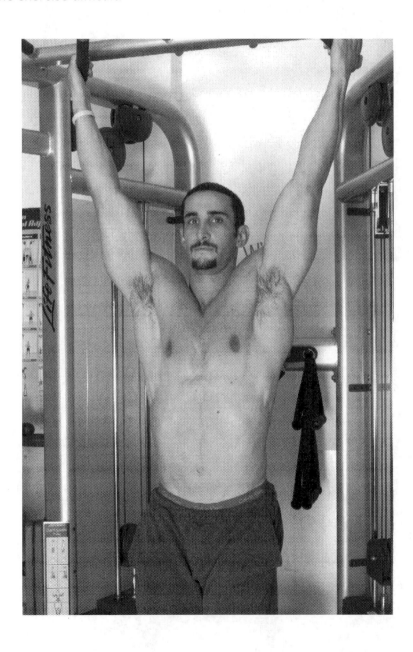

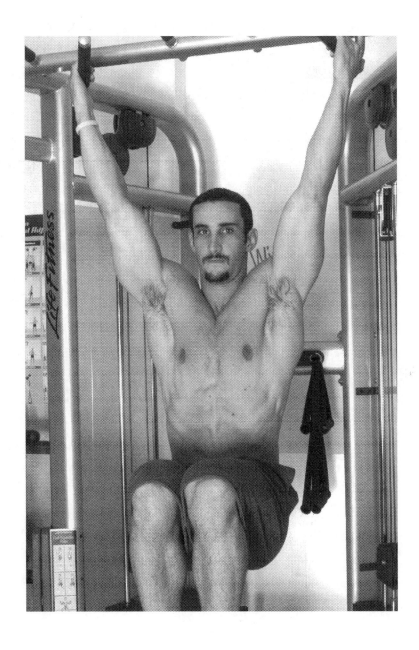

Machine Crunches – not so much of a fan of machines but I need to make mention of them. They are ok to use for those who hate the floor or just want a variety of options. They tend to place more stress on the lower back than the actual abdominal region. If you can master the art of crunches then any machine should suffice since you will know how to perform a proper repetition, breathe gracefully and contract to your absolute maximum potential.

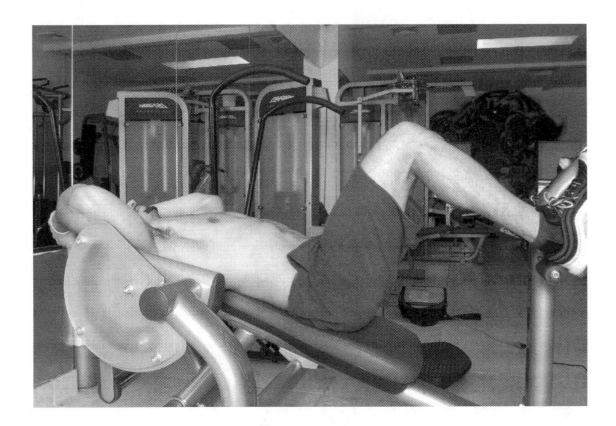

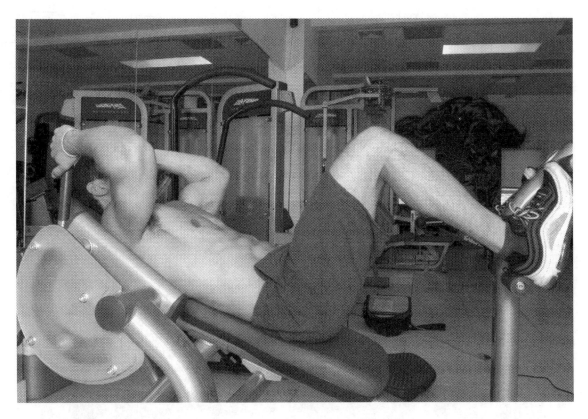

Make sure that when using any abdominal machine that you're using only the abdominal muscle. Avoid getting help from your lower back, your biceps or any other muscle. Perform every repetition controlled and properly.

Leg Raises – this can be done on either the floor or a bench (can be a flat bench or an adjustable bench). Lie on your back with your hands behind your butt and legs extended straight out. Keeping your legs straight begin to raise them as high as you can without lifting your back off the bench or floor, then lower them half an inch off the floor. By keeping your legs straight out and half an inch off the floor will help keep the muscle contracted and assure that you are using proper form. I see many people do leg raises and lower their legs till it hits the floor so that they can create some sort of momentum – avoid this mistake. I also mentioned you can use an adjustable bench because while on an incline, the stress on the abdominals is tougher and hits the lower portion while developing core strength and an overall tighter mid-section.

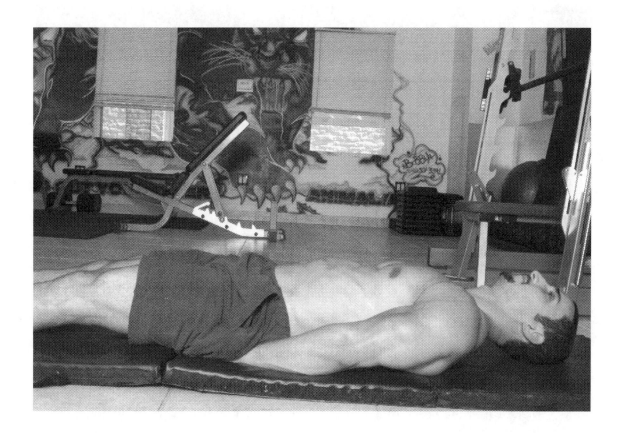

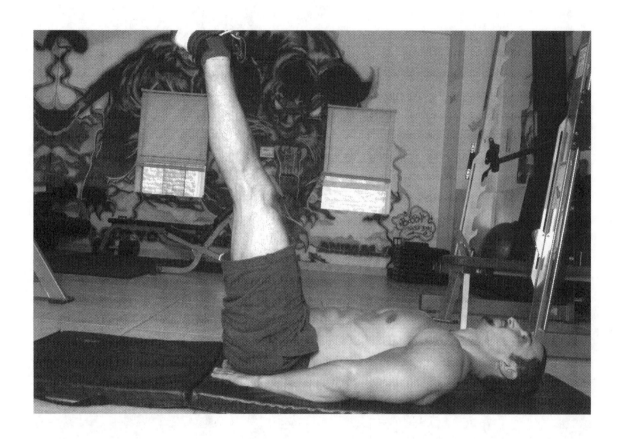

Leg Tucks – seated on a bench or on the floor – if proper form and contraction is reached then this exercise serves well for developing both the upper and lower abdominals.

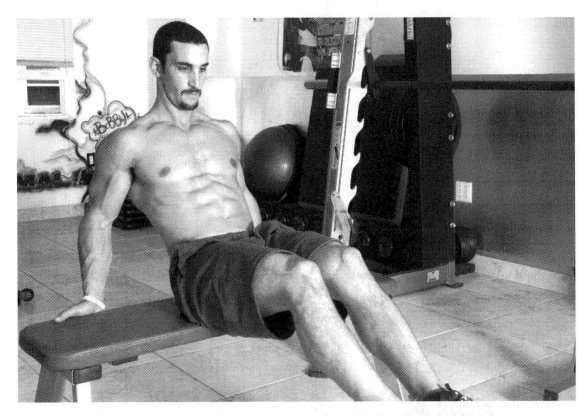

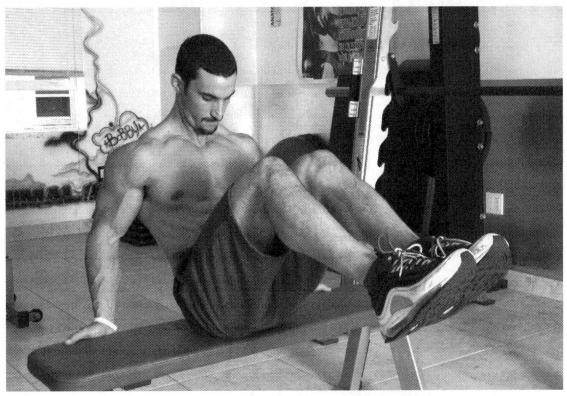

You can also do this exercise to trigger the obliques by doing it to the side.

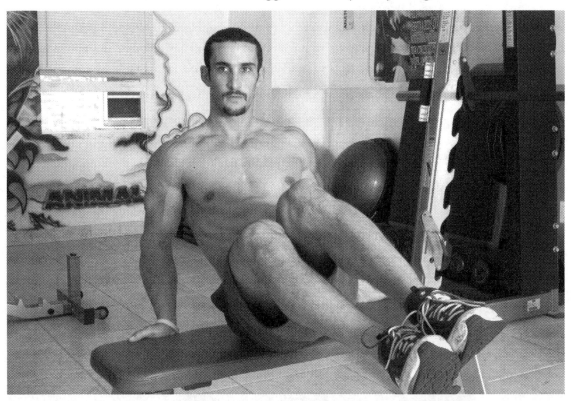

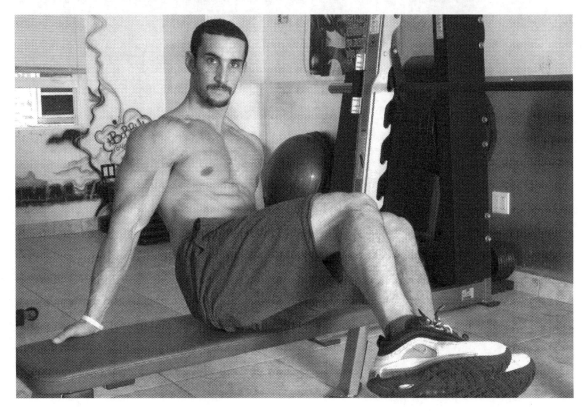

Sit-Up's – I am not a big fan of this exercise but I felt I had to mention it. Sit-up's, at least I believe, works the abs slightly in its beginning phase then it shifts that stress and tension into the lower back. When I work out my abs I only want my abs to be worked and no other body part. I have a strong lower back but I save that for a separate day and a separate routine. Many people suffer from severe or chronic back pains so as a trainer I don't usually have them perform it. However, once in a while you get your share of either boxers or young children who are resilient and can endure these sit-up's. I see them do this exercise with ease and they go for a good amount of time. I guess it works for them. Like I always say – what works for you, might not work for others and vice versa. Always do what you think works for you. The only true expert in determining what exercises work is YOU.

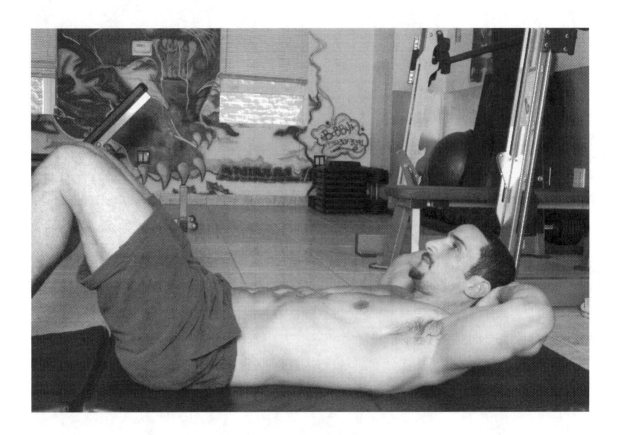

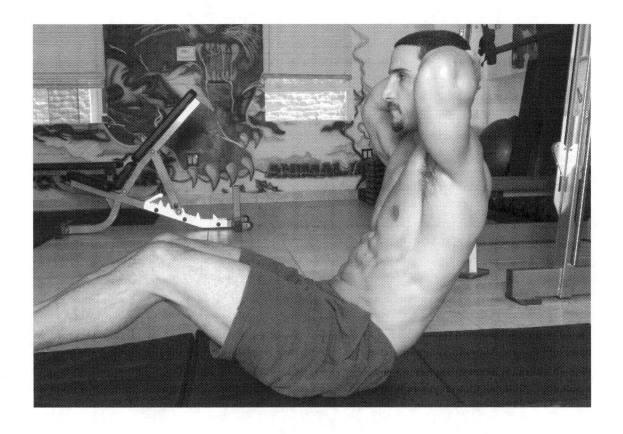

Leg Raises on a Dip Station or Vertical Bench – this is similar to hanging leg raises with the exception that your back is now supported against a pad. You are not hanging on a bar and your arms are actually supported on the bench. Make sure your body and back are steady while performing the exercise. You can either bend your knees or keep your legs straight out. Both ways you need to make sure you are flexing your abs through the full range of motion.

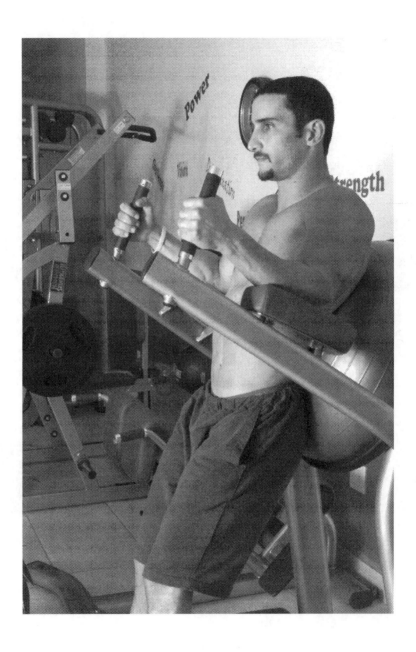

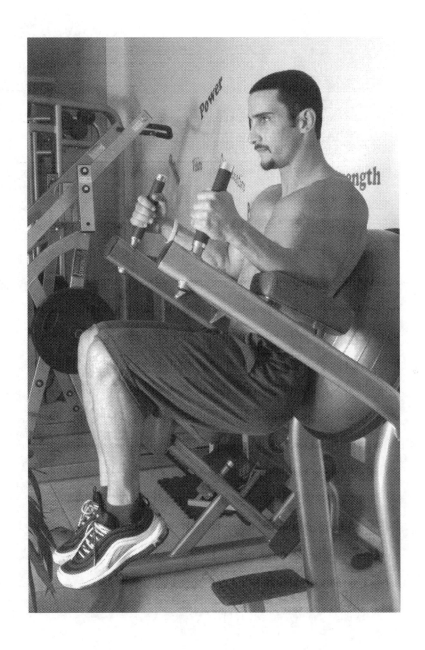

Plank (usually done on your elbows and toes) – lie face down on the floor or mat while resting on your forearms, elbows and toes. Make sure your back is flat and parallel to the floor. Slightly tilt your pelvis and contract your abdominals so that you prevent your rear end from sticking up in the air. Hold yourself in this position for as long as you can (20-60 seconds) and try to repeat it for at least 5 reps or so.

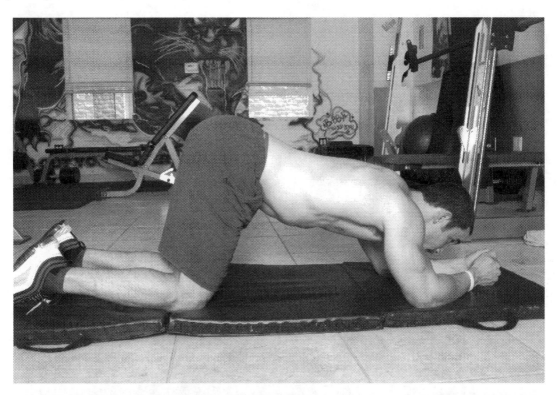

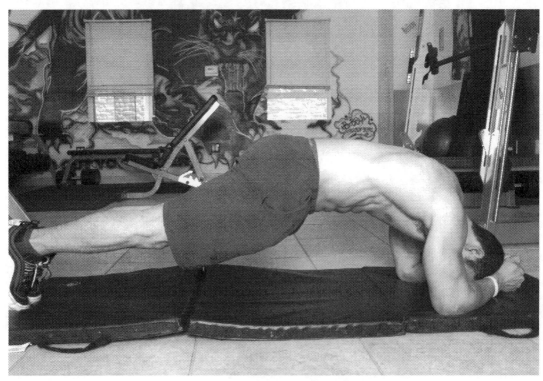

Make sure that your stomach is being squeezed to ensure maximum contractions. If this becomes easy for you then have your partner or someone place a ball (physioball or medicine ball) on the lower portion of your back and apply pressure. Try to resist the tension and hold the same position for a few seconds.

With the recent awareness in fitness many physioballs, kettle bells and balls, medicine balls, foam rollers, and plenty more such items have become popular. They are excellent for resistance, stretching, balance, control, stability and coordination and can be used for almost every exercise and body part. They are extremely popular in aerobic classes and definitely great for all sorts of ab exercises. Like I said and will continue to say, variety in exercises, equipment and even these BALLS can be beneficial to your goals and your needs. There are so many other exercises for the abdominals but once again I listed the most common and most used exercises. I see so many people experimenting with benches, cables and machines all the time and yet none are close to the results you get from the basic exercises. These exercises were done for years before fancy gyms came about and before people were developing fancy machines and contraptions. They are the basics and the foundation to all newly innovated exercises. I encourage you to experiment and try all new exercises your body can handle and your mind can conceive. Make sure you know how to execute the basics perfectly and properly before you start embarking on these new venues. Once you can control form and proper movements you can do almost anything. Before you learned how to run and play, I am sure that your parents taught you how to walk and even fall so that you can pick yourself up and try again.

Before I completely end this chapter I would like to leave you with a few routines for working the obliques. A lot of the oblique's deals with your genetic make-up but it can't hurt giving these exercises a try.

Windshield Wipers

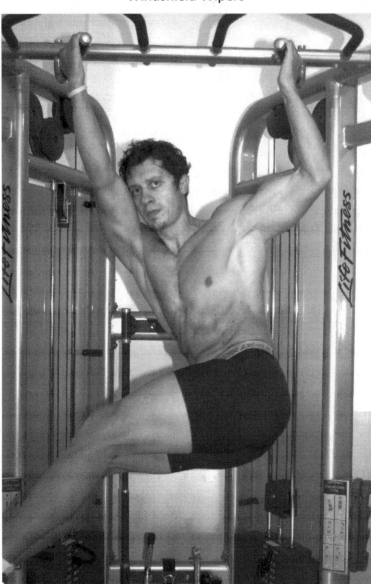

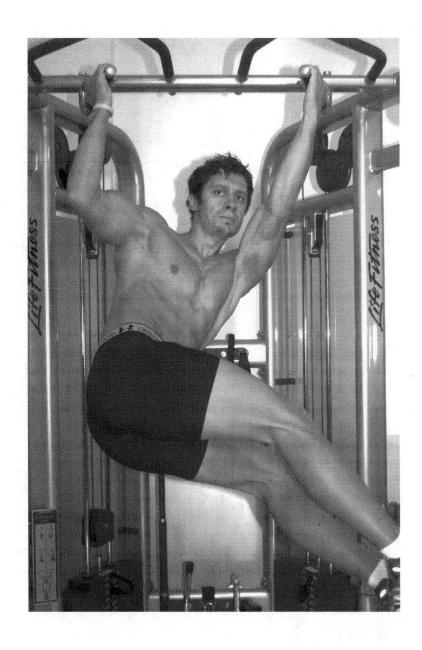

Twist Crunches on a Decline Bench

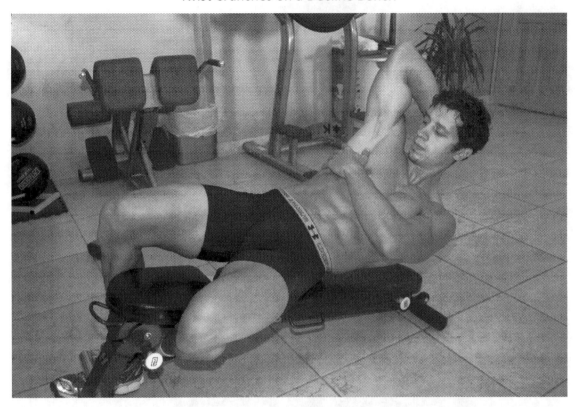

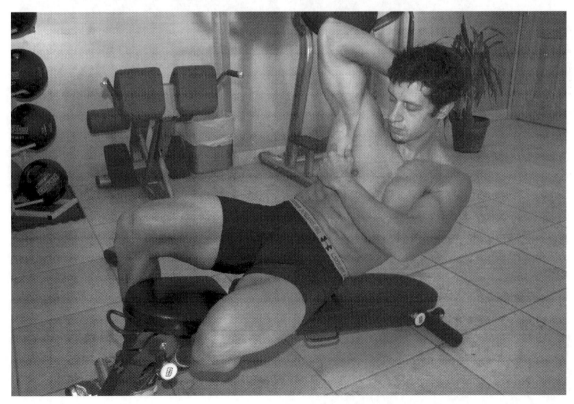

Side Crunches on the Hyperextension Machine

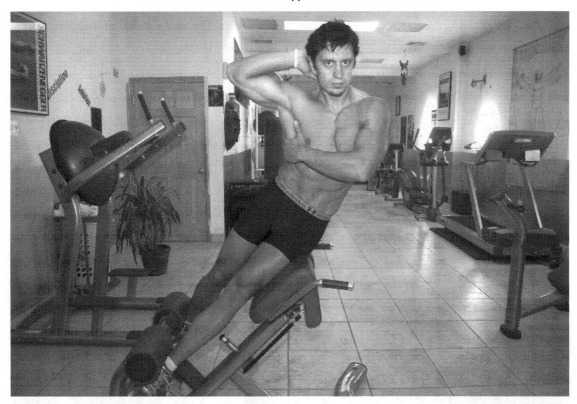

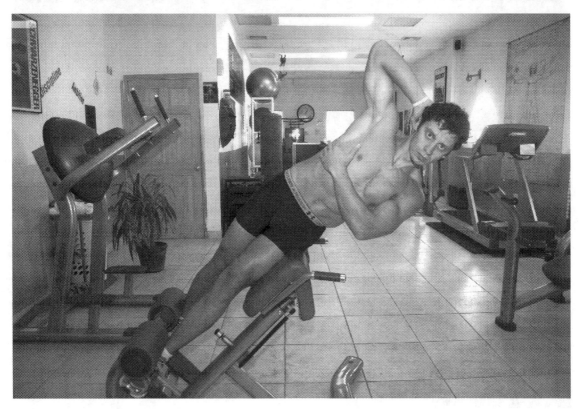

Side Crunches on a mat (you need a partner to hold you down for this particular exercise. Not very common but extremely effective)

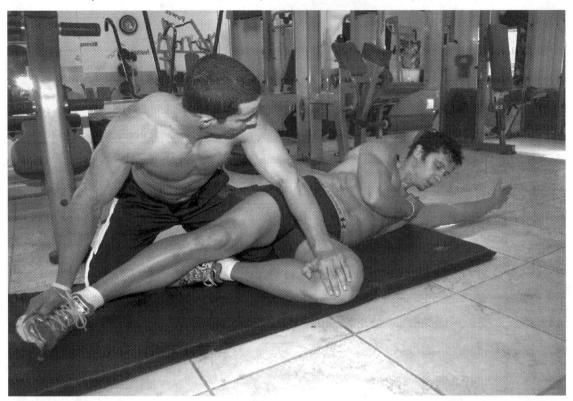

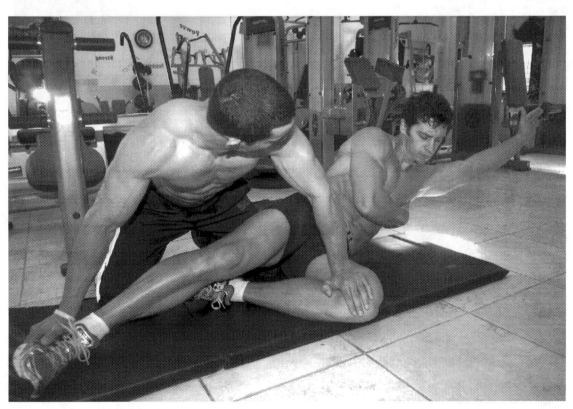

Standing Oblique Crunches with a medicine ball (you can also use a dumbbell or a free weight)

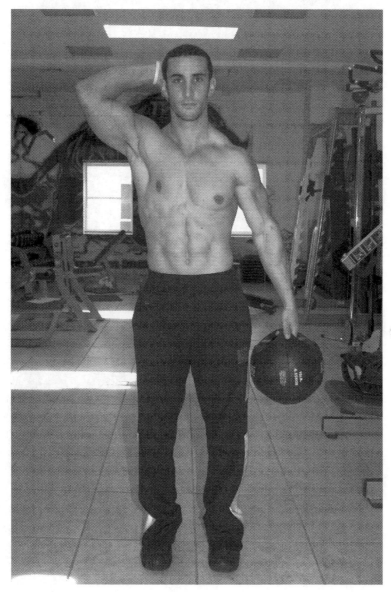

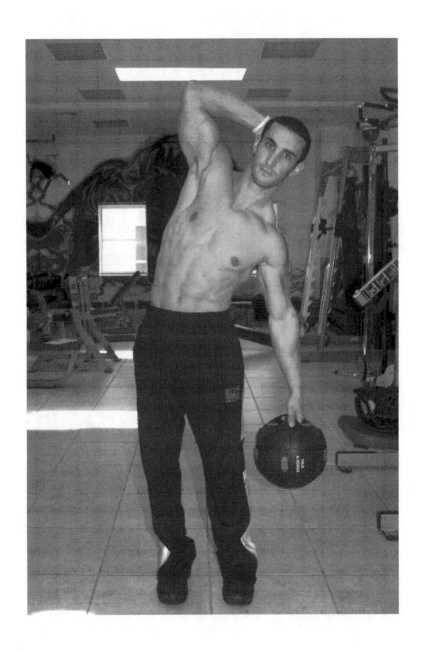

Chapter 9
Who Am I? More Basic Jargon

Fitness is a great sport and can easily be suited for every person, every body type, every sex, every color, every race and every age. What makes it all interesting is that we all have different physical characteristics. Some of us are taller, shorter, smaller, wider, narrower, lighter or darker, have different levels of endurance, blood cells, muscle cells and fat cells. So I ask you the important question, who are you? Now I know this is a broad question but I refer to it in terms of body type. There are three fundamentally different physical body types: Ectomorph, Mesomorph, and Endomorph. According to The New Encyclopedia of Modern Day Bodybuilding, Arnold describes these types as the following:

Ectomorph – characterized by a short upper body, long arms and legs, long narrow feet and hands, and very little fat storage; narrowness in the chest and shoulders, with generally long, thin muscles.

Mesomorph – characterized by a large chest, long torso, solid muscle structure, and great strength

Endomorph – characterized by a soft musculature, round face, short neck, wide hips, and heavy fat storage.

Now of course no one fits the above descriptions down to a science. Many people can be a combination of all three but the foundation needs to be established. Since every individual is blessed with a different body type then we have to determine that every type responds differently to training. Remember, I always said that what works for one person may not necessarily work for another. Any one of the three body types can be developed, but only through proper training and nutrition. I can assure you that once you understand your body type, you can have a clear sense as to what exercises and what style of training works best for you. All it takes is a sense of knowledge and understanding and you can easily be on your way with no frustration, hesitation or excuses. In short I can break it down for you as easy as I can: An Ectomorph's main objectives are to gain muscle weight (become more massive). Most of the muscle mass will come from heavy training and enough food in terms of protein and carbohydrates. Since the mesomorph is kind of an in between body type then having a sound nutritional program along with a variety of exercises is vital. You already have the frame so now you have to sculpt it to your likening. Endomorph is similar to mesomorph in that it is easy to build muscle and put on some mass. However, they have to be careful from gaining weight so diet is crucial - maybe a low-caloric diet with proper supplementation. If you're an endomorph make sure you are getting a minimum or just exact amount of protein, carbohydrates and fats, otherwise if you're having more than the minimum amount you will begin to gain fat and weight.

So now that we found out our body type and went over a great amount of exercises, let's discuss some basic principles to weight training. Once we establish these laws, as I call them, then I think we are ready to go over a list of workout programs. I am sure that while reading this book you wrote some stuff down and probably even asked somebody what the hell is a superset. What does Kobi mean when he says Drop Set? What do you actually mean when you make reference to Isolation training? Well strap in and begin to take notes, or just memorize these principles. I can assure you that most people don't even know the technical names but now you will.

The Shocking Principle – as its name implies – you totally shock your body by constantly changing around routines, exercises and other aspects of your workout. Since the body is an amazing phenomenon and very adaptable, it can easily get accustomed to workouts, movements and other things related to working out. Therefore, if you always work out the same without changes or even put the same amount of stress on the body, chances are you will not see the results you expected. The shocking principle allows you change various techniques in your training, such as: (1) using more or less weight (2) changing the amount of repetitions and sets (3) speeding up your workouts (4) cutting down your rest in between sets and exercises (5) changing your routines and exercises periodically – for example you can change the order in which you perform the exercises. Start with the last exercise first and jumble around other exercises in between. (6) Do some unfamiliar exercises – in other words try something new.

The next two principles require you to (but don't have to) work out with a training partner. I started my career working out with a partner for the mere fact that he was more experienced than me. I was kind of like an apprentice just eager to learn and have my chance to shine. Scottie, my training partner, would always push me and encourage me. Positive feedback and gratification were so important in my early stages of development. Weight training is a strenuous activity/hobby and having someone else by your side enduring it is not only a relief but a big burden off your shoulders. We constantly challenged our bodies and ourselves by never allowing the other to fail. We developed a mutual understanding and built upon that – we always knew what the other person was thinking and a bond was formed. This person became a true friend because he cared about my overall performance, physique, health and most importantly me. In return so did I. We trained so hard and competed in numerous natural bodybuilding competitions as one. We strived for excellence and we fought through tough and brutal workouts. The best thing about my training partner was that we had the same goals and a competitive edge. We always tried to outlift one another just to create an atmosphere that catered to incredible and unforeseen results. We never competed against one another but rather competed as a team to see one another grow. So I cannot stress the importance of choosing a workout partner that you can trust and learn from. So with that all said and done the next two principles are Forced Repetitions and Partial Repetitions.

Forced Repetitions – as its name applies, is a method of forcing out additional reps once your set is about complete. Your workout partner will be right by your side supplying you extra attention and assistance so that you can force these last two or three reps out. For example, let's say you are doing a set of flat bench presses with a heavy weight, or even a light weight at that, for a set of 10 repetitions. Since your mind has already determined the number of reps you're most likely to stop once you reach for whatever reason. With your training partner in back of you yelling and screaming he will begin to notice the moment you are exhausted and gradually help you pump out two or three more forced reps. This method forces your body to work overtime and call for more recruitment of muscle fibers to tear. You can't believe the pump you get from just doing an extra few of these forced reps. You're adrenaline levels are now sky high and you say to yourself wow I want to try this again and again and again.

Partial Repetitions – These are similar to forced repetitions except for the fact that you are doing partial reps. With forced reps you still complete a full range of motion with the help of your partner. Partial reps you just keep some tension on the muscle by doing exactly what this method requires – a partial rep. A good example of this is the preacher curl. You start off by doing your complete set of whatever number of reps, getting a full range of motion and ensuring proper form throughout. Once your muscles become fatigued and exhausted and you have no more energy or power left you lift the bar to the top of the motion and lower it even just a few inches or degrees for a good amount of repetitions. This totally shocks and burns the bicep muscle and is highly effective and a great way to get that pump.

Isolation principle – This is really a more informative principle than anything. Once you learn the basics of working out and all the different exercises you can then properly understand this philosophy. You have to be able to do exactly what this principle states, and that is isolate body parts by using various isolation exercises. What is an isolation exercise? Good question and the answer is simple – it's an exercise that only places stress on a muscle group or even just part of a muscle. Your muscles have something known as stabilizers. These stabilizers help your body either push or pull and complete an exercise. A common exercise that we see the stabilizers work greatly is the bench press. How many times have you done a bench press and either felt it in your shoulders (deltoids), triceps or even forearms and lower back. The answer is plenty of times – this is because since one part of the body is either weak or behind in strength and development so it draws help from these stabilizer muscles to better aid you. The isolation principle calls for specific exercises that target one muscle group and one muscle group only. With the case of chest, you can perform DB Fly's to maximize the Pecs and isolate them without any help from other body parts. So I mentioned that once you understand your body, your physique and your knowledge of weight training, then you will see how important this principle really is.

Weak point Training or Priority Principle – everyone, and I mean everyone, has some point of their body that is either not developed or even overdeveloped. No one has the perfect physique or body – that's not the way God made us or otherwise we will all be in trouble. Instead we need to pay close attention to the basics and the appreciation for absolute proportion. Everybody I know always mentioned to me that they just want their body to be in proportion. So this principle allows you to analyze your physique and take notes as to what you need to pay close attention to. Some body types can develop better and faster than others, while others are credited to poor or rich genetics. Once you understand what needs to be done then go ahead and begin training effectively on that body part. Schedule a twice-a-week routine maybe, where you attack that muscle or muscles twice a week for example. Develop a workout that you know will work for you – specific workouts for every body part is attainable no matter the development you are looking for. Just remember, if a body part is not responding for whatever reason, don't just be quick to give up and accept it as a fact. Do something about it and look for a solution – there is always an answer and the answer is applying this priority principle.

Supersets – I have made numerous references to this word and so now we need to go into details. Supersets are two continuance exercises performed in a row without resting or stopping. This requires a good amount of endurance and is highly effective. You can superset either the same body part (Chest & Chest) or two different body parts (Chest & Back). Performing supersets within the same muscle group allows you to pound and absolutely demolish away that muscle group. A good example for supersetting within the same muscle group is: Flat Bench Presses superset with Flat Dumbbell Fly's.

While Supersetting two different body parts, this allows one muscle to rest while the other is being worked. An example of this is working out the triceps and biceps. Both are great for endurance and for a sick pump and there is no right or wrong answer. The best way to establish which one works best for you is to just try it. Go into the gym and one day try to perform two exercises back to back for the same body part and another day for two different body parts. I always like to use supersets for training the same muscle group because of the tremendous pump I get. I feel like my body explodes rapidly and almost nothing can stop me. Amazing what these supersets can do to the performance of the exercises and results.

The Stripping or Drop-Set Method – This means that you reduce the weight you are using for a particular exercise to enable yourself to get more repetitions and a burning sensation. If you begin to see that the weight you are using is too heavy to continue don't just stop and relax, lower the weight and continue to bang out some more quality repetitions. It doesn't mean that your muscles are totally fatigued; it only means that they can't endure any more of a certain weight so lowering the weight can be beneficial to you. Your body will work harder and more muscle recruitment will be needed for you to complete the descending weight. This method can be used for almost every exercise and muscle group. You can apply this to all plate-loaded machines or weighted plates for barbells. There is also no set guide for how many times you can drop – just make sure it's not too light and easy to lift so that you don't burn out or just complete a dead set. A good example of this is doing Lat pull downs: Since this exercise is performed on a machine with a plate stack you can drop weight at different intervals. If you start with 150 pounds and get 6 reps, drop it to 120 and attempt 8-10 reps, then drop it again to 90 pounds for 12-15 reps. This is a three way drop and it consists of 30 pound decreases and believe it or not in that one exercise you did approximately 26 repetitions. You got your set for strength and power and then for definition while at the same time getting endurance levels to increase. There are so many exercises and ways you can apply this stripping method so don't be afraid to work with trial and error.

Run-the-Rack Method – this is a form of drop-setting or stripping method except it only deals with dumbbells. It is called running-the-rack because the rack is where the dumbbells are stationed and that's where you will be for these exercises. You can do all sorts of exercises and is highly effective with biceps and deltoids. If you are doing lateral raises this will work just fine. You begin with the heaviest weight you can handle using good form and drop down 5 pounds every set without rest. So I start off with 35 pound dumbbells and work my own down to 15 pounds – yes this is insane and highly demanding. Once you determine what your ideal heaviest weight is then you should be ready to go. You will need to push and constantly strive for completion. It burns, it's hard and yes extremely challenging but then again other things in life are harder. Once you complete the decrease in weight that is considered one set and not 5 or 6. Try doing this 4 times and see how fatigued you become. It is also a bit time consuming so assure that you're keeping good form throughout rather than rushing and either cheating or not doing the movement properly.

Circuit Training – this is a routine where you do a full body workout in one day. You pick some basic exercises and perform a few sets on one body part and continue to other body parts. It is a routine that requires little rest and usually completed quickly. For each body part you perform two or three exercises doing high repetitions. These exercises are basic and you can mix between machines and free weights. It's a good way to get a pump but it should not be done daily or weekly. Circuits are used for those who are beginners, those who have limited time and those who both came back from an injury or rehabilitation and need a way to stay active and mobile. It is not challenging or stressful since you are working out lightly and is perfect for an occasional shocking of the muscles.

The Pre-exhaust Principle – this is a challenging principle and not really used much in today's world of fitness. Most of us that work out always like to start working out with the powerful exercises first and work our way towards the easier and less strenuous movements last. Since we feel fresh and strong in the early going of our workouts, we tend to utilize this strength and lift heavy for the first two exercises or so. Well this principle requires you doing the exact opposite. Begin with the most basic routines that don't require heavy weight and work your way from there. What does this mean? Well a prime example of this principle works well with shoulders. You start off with lateral DB Raises or Frontal Raises, or Upright Rows or Arnold Presses and continue with this pattern. By the third or fourth exercise your shoulders should be fatigued and completely exhausted. Just as you think your shoulders cannot endure any more pounding you are dead wrong. Let's say your last exercise is going to be DB shoulders presses or barbell presses or any other power movement. So then you must work a drop harder to complete the exercise. Your body will need to recruit more muscle fiber and use the help of stabilizers to help you complete every repetition and every set. This is another great way to shock the body and see results more rapidly. I still find myself using this principle quite often and definitely enjoy the challenge of completing the workouts while being totally exhausted.

The I-Go-You-Go Method – this method is one of my other absolute favors and requires you to have a training partner. This particular method is great for shocking your muscles and doing every set or repetition with great intensity. You and your training partner immediately hand over the weight to the other while never putting the weight down. Sounds a bit complicated? A good explanation of this technique works great with the biceps while performing barbell curls. While doing these curls and facing one another you hand the barbell to the your partner after completing a set and just waiting till he hands it back to you. It is like a back and forth cycle for the duration and leaves you feeling painful and sore. You can both do the curls to failure while handing it off to each other, setting a particular number of repetitions and going till those repetitions get less and less or choosing a time to determine how long you will be performing these curls. I tried all three ways and they are all productive. The basic idea of this technique is that you go when it's your turn regarding how tired you are getting and whether or not you are ready. The degree of intensity you can get with this method is phenomenal. The I-Go-You-Go method is designed strictly for training smaller muscles like biceps, triceps and calves. Other body parts require way too much energy and demand that chances are you will run out of steam quickly. Arnold Schwarzenegger was a huge fan of this method and used it for biceps training with his partners.

Negative Repetitions – whenever you lift a weight in a controlled and contractile motion you perform what is defined as a positive movement. When you lower the weight and extend the working muscle you perform what is called the negative movement. Negative repetitions are great for placing stress on the muscles and creating a great burning sensation. To get the full benefit of negatives in your everyday workouts, always lower the weights slowly and under control. Make believe as if there is some type of resistance on your way down, rather than letting the weight drop. You want to actually work hard on these negatives and maintain the same pace and consistency throughout each rep and each set. To make things a bit challenging, at the end of a set when your muscles are fatigued, lift the weight up to its ending position and hold it for approximately 10-15 seconds before lowering them. For example, when performing a set of dumbbell lateral raises at the end of your set keep the dumbbells with arms fully extended and just hold for as long as you can. Your arms should begin to shake and your shoulders should begin to burn tremendously. Try it!

The Rule of Ten's (10) or The Power of Ten (P.O.T) – this is a routine that I designed for my biceps and triceps workouts on days off when I wanted a great pump. I start off by a cable station and stay there for the duration of the workout, which happens to be 10 minutes. What kind of workout can you possibly get in 10 minutes is what you are thinking? Well this is a great workout that will have your arms burning and screaming for more. You pick four exercises utilizing different cable attachments, resting 10 seconds after every set and exercise and should be completed in 10 minutes. Thus, make sure you stay where you are at all times and limit your distractions (water break, conversation, etc...). I enjoy this particular workout because it leads to a great accumulation of blood and lactic acid in the arms and creates an ultimate pump. Here are two workouts that I enjoy for the triceps and biceps. Make sure your rest is exactly 10 seconds and be quick when changing exercises and cable attachments. Remember, every second counts. I use this technique quite often with my clients and all absolutely love it and are overwhelmed at the pump they get. They are just baffled as to how a 10 minute routine can be so effective. Remember, you are doing 4 exercises in 10 minutes totaling 160 repetitions (4 sets of 10 repetitions X 4 exercises = 160). Just give this a try and see what happens! If you are daring and love challenges then try to apply this for other body parts.

Here is an example of how the P.O.T method should be applied for an arm workout.

Triceps	Biceps
Rope Pressdowns	Wide-Grip Bar Cable Curls
Over-head Rope Extensions	Close-Grip Bar Cable Curls
Straight Bar Pressdowns	Reverse Grip Cable Curls (any bar)
V-Bar Pressdowns	Rope Hammer Curls

Chapter 10
Workout Routines – What Do I Do and How Do I Know What to Do and When to Do? An Explanation of all Your Dues - Do's.

I have listed many exercises through these chapters and a detailed explanation to them as well. If you read through this book thoroughly your mind should have became aroused and curious as to what you need to do in the gym. Weight training is a science in the sense that you are the mad scientist trying to figure out what works best for you. You spend numerous days and nights reading about fitness and then experimenting what you have just read and saw. Now you begin to ask yourself what routines, programs and exercises should I be doing? So the only answer I have is to start from a beginner level and work your way up to advanced or even master levels. There is no precise answer set in stone for what you need to do and how you need to do it. However, the most logical answer I can think of is Rome was not built in a day, and I am even quite sure that mistakes and horrific events were made, but the end result was a masterpiece. A true work of art, innovation, expertise, hard work and vision was put into Rome. Your body is kind of similar in the sense that the same attitude and characteristics are needed for every aspect of fitness and healthy living. You have your basic rules and principles, all which are great for leading you into the right direction so why not continue to build on that and create your masterpiece.

In this chapter, I will give you a basic formula for how you can design your routines and programs. I will review many different routines and exercises and sort of guide you in a calculated direction. The basics you already have just from reading this book, so I will include a list of all the ingredients you need to bake something interesting. No we are not baking cakes, rather we are baking the ingredients needed to create the new "YOU." Since there are numerous amounts of body parts and only 7 days in the week we have to be precise and make sure that each body part is being worked on effectively. In general, or most often, we work out larger muscle groups before smaller muscle groups. This allows us to work the larger muscles thoroughly and accurately. Remember, there is no set order to work out but from my own, and so many others experience, larger muscles first and smaller muscles last. Also, try to keep the sequence of a workout in order – you do this by separating your body into two zones or spheres – upper body and lower body. I usually tend to train upper body parts alone and allowing for lower body (legs) to be trained all alone with no stress on any other muscle group. Just remember whatever your goals are try to dedicate a good amount of time for exercise and recovery. You must approach every workout with a clear vision and an all-out effort to actually see results. The amount of work and dedication you put into fitness will dictate how your overall appearance and attitude will suddenly look and change.

Now that you are almost ready to go over a routine, I need to list a few more important pieces of information. After any workout allow your body to recuperate at least 24-48 hours before you can work out that body part again. Unless, your body is so quick in repairing itself and you are getting both enough sleep and proper supplementation (protein) then this need not apply to you. Try to avoid working out seven continuous and consistent days and allow your body to recover appropriately. A four or 5 day routine is fine but just make sure that you are allowing one day rest in between to break things up. Trust me your body will thank you for that rest day and it will repay you in more ways than you can imagine. Ok so we have to go over a few more details before we can begin. Each individual should have an idea as to what their goals are, what their schedule looks like and the amount of days they can dedicate. Your goals will dictate how much time and effort you need to spend in the gym or fitness facility. If you have a trainer, as mentioned earlier, tell them what your goals are and let them design a program. Your goals, needs and desires should be realistic and attainable. A few common goals I hear often are: (1) Improve my health – this includes improving core strength, working on posture and endurance levels and a few others (2) Change my looks completely (body wise) (3) Interested in training for an athletic event and (4) Just want girls/guys to start noticing me. Significantly changing any of these goals requires time commitment and a true passion for achieving results. You will need to endure a good amount of pain - gym related, tasteless diets and even many grueling workouts. But in the end you will be standing notoriously and victoriously and no one can ever take that away from you. You earned it!

- By the way, don't expect to look like all those fitness people you see on infomercials and countless models on TV and magazines. No one knows what they endured and no one can be certain that they did it the way I am preaching. There are plenty of surgeries, drugs and other such horrible things, which I don't even want to mention, that people have taken to look the way they look. Everyone is always looking for the easy way out – the quickest fix. Well this is not the case with me and my book. It is a passion and a yearning that I have for the wonderful world of fitness. I can't describe the feeling I still get when I walk into a gym. It is the absolute highlight of my day; it makes me so much more focused and leaves me with a great feeling of accomplishment. Just keep in mind that healthy living is at its absolute highest point and many people are becoming more physically fit and living longer. It truly is a necessity and should be treated as a valuable asset. After all, YOUR MOST VALUABLE ASSET OR POSSESSION IS YOU. That is why I coined the saying, "Fitness is not a luxury, it is a necessity."

Part I – Beginner Basic Routine/Program

If you're a beginner, then pay close attention to these programs and don't go jumping right into a more difficult program. Whatever your friend is doing or whatever you read in a magazine can wait until you think you are fully accustomed to all basic movements, proper form and understanding of your mission. You start out with light weights and relatively few exercises and then gradually build on your routines. Usually a three day routine works perfect for beginners – a great routine is an every other day routine (Monday, Wednesday, Friday or Tuesday, Thursday, Sunday). For easier understanding, I will just label these days as workout #1, #2 and #3 and you can decide what days work best for you.

<u>Workout #1 – Chest & Triceps</u>

Flat-Bench Dumbbell Presses – 4 sets of 15 repetitions (try to keep a moderate weight that allows you to perform 4 sets with proper form). I like for beginners to start with dumbbells so that they learn how to work each arm independently and allows for the use of coordination and stability.

Incline Dumbbell Presses – 4 sets of 15 repetitions (the same rules apply for this as mentioned with Flat DB Presses)

Pec-Dec Fly's or Machine fly's – 4 sets of 15 repetitions and you can try to increase the weight a little so that it becomes challenging.

Push-Up's – end off your chest routine with some push-up's – do one set and see how many you can get and repeat for two or three sets.

Rope Press downs – 4 sets of 15 repetitions with at least 20-30 second rest in between sets

Kickbacks (using a dumbbell) – 4 sets of 15 repetitions at a moderate weight (in order to get best results you need to use a light weight to ensure proper form)

Bench Dips – 4 sets of 15 repetitions with a 20 second rest in between sets. Make sure that at the end of the movement you lock your elbows and hold for a second or two before doing another repetition.

OR

Flat DB Presses – 4 sets of 15 repetitions

Flat Barbell Presses – 4 sets of 15 repetitions

Flat DB Fly's – 4 sets of 15 repetitions

Any Chest Machine – 3 sets of 12 repetitions (since machines are easier to handle – increase the weight after every set within moderation. Don't try the big boy routine just yet.

V-Bar Press downs – 4 sets of 15 repetitions (make sure you are getting a full range of motion and a good contraction)

Rope Press downs – 4 sets of 15 repetitions

Skull-Crushers using dumbbells – 4 sets of 12 repetitions – make sure your elbows are in place and not flaring out when lowering the dumbbells to your fore head.

Workout #2 – Back & Biceps

Wide-grip lat Pull downs – 4 sets of 15 repetitions

Close-grip Lat Pull downs – 4 sets of 15 repetitions

Machine Rows (either a machine or Hammer Strength) – 4 sets of 12 repetitions (increase the weight slightly if you can, but you don't have to.

Hyperextensions – 3 sets of 15 repetitions – try to get a full range of motion

Seated Alternate DB Curls – 3 sets of 15 repetitions – doing this seated will not allow you to cheat or get support from your lower back

Wide-Grip Cable Curls – (use an e-z bar attachment) – 3 sets of 15 repetitions – make sure you get a full range of motion and a good contraction

Dumbbell Hammer Curls – 3 sets of 15 repetitions

OR

Pull-Up's – 3 sets of 10 repetitions (this is challenging and requires upper body strength and endurance)

Wide-Grip Lat Pull downs – 4 sets of 15, 15, 12, 12 repetitions (increase the weight)

One-Arm DB Rows – 3 sets of 15 repetitions

Hyperextensions – 4 sets of 15 repetitions

Alternate DB Curls – 4 sets of 25 repetitions – yes you are going to get a total of 100 repetitions

Barbell Curls – 4 sets of 15 repetitions

Hammer Curls – 3 sets of 12 repetitions (keep the weight constant)

Workout #3 – Legs & Shoulders

Leg Extensions – 4 sets of 20 repetitions with a one second hold at the top of the exercise (use a good weight since this can be a bit challenging)

Lunges – for those who need help with coordination and balance then you should perform stationary lunges. That is where one leg is being worked while the other is bending. However, for those with coordination and stability you can perform alternate lunges. This exercise can be done with either a weighted bar, dumbbells at your side or no weight at all. Try to get 3 sets of 15 repetitions

Squats – 4 sets of 15 repetitions using a normal toe slightly out position. Once again this can be done with either a barbell over your neck or dumbbells held at your side. If that's challenging for you then begin doing squats without any weight except your own body weight.

Lateral Dumbbell Raises – 4 sets of 15 repetitions (keep a moderate weight and rest 30 seconds in between every set)

Front Dumbbell Raises – 4 sets of 15 repetitions (keep a moderate weight and rest 30 seconds in between every set)

Shoulder Dumbbell Presses – 4 sets of 12 repetitions (if you want you can increase the weight very slightly to ensure proper range of motion)

Dumbbell Shrugs – 3 sets of 15 repetitions – make sure you get a full contraction at the top of the movement. In other words, bring the dumbbells as high as you can (making believe you can touch your ears)

OR

Leg Presses – 4 sets of 15 repetitions

Lunges – 4 sets of 15 repetitions

Leg extensions – 4 sets of 15 repetitions

Leg Curls – 4 sets of 15 repetitions

Arnold Presses – 4 sets of 15 repetitions

Dumbbell Lateral Raises – 4 sets of 15 repetitions

Reverse Pec-Dec Fly's – 3 sets of 20 repetitions

Smith Machine Shrugs – 4 sets of 12 repetitions – try to increase the weight after every set

So for the Beginner workouts we went over the three common routines and exercises. A 45 minute routine is sufficient for all beginners until they can get acclimated to different workouts. This every other day routine is common and allows the body to properly rest and recuperate. I like the whole idea of high repetitions with multiple sets for a tremendous pump with both a great sweat and heavy breathing. Your main objectives as a beginner are to learn:

- Coordination

- Build Endurance & Strength

- Improve breathing skills

- Learn and improve stability, control and agility

- Form and posture – two vital elements to master so that once you pass the beginner level you can easily adapt to different exercises and routines (he who controls form, can later control weight)

Part II - Intermediate Routines/Programs

For those who have experience working out and know their share of exercises, this chapter is ideal for you. The intermediate level is obviously more challenging than the beginner level, but is a bit more fun. I say it's fun because the basics are now behind you and you can begin to experiment slightly with new machines and equipment and increase your weight in certain exercises. It is a bit less regimental and boring as the beginner level but also can be a bit more challenging for others. The intermediate level also dictates your performance and your true desire for fitness. If you begin to enjoy it and appreciate it at the beginner level then chances are you will climb the ladder much quicker than those who are still dealing with certain issues. These issues can be lack of motivation, slow to adapt, no desire to continue and also lack of knowledge regarding weight training. If you enjoy it then I am quite sure you will also educate yourself on it so that you can pursue that ultimate body. The more you learn and read, the more you will benefit. So with that all said and done let's list a few of my favorite routines. Be prepared to be challenged but also be prepared to have some fun and excitement. You will see how strong your body is and how certain things you never believed were possible now become reality. Once again I will design two workouts for every body part and allow you to mix and match to fit your schedule. At the intermediate level at least four days are possible for weight training so that you can maximize all your potential on each body part.

In the beginner level workouts I went with a basic routine that focused on two pushing body parts and two pulling body parts or muscles. This type of split allows you to work two muscles without using any other muscle groups. If I lost many of you on this area then allow me to explain. Chest exercises are considered to be a pushing motion; so are the triceps. The back and the biceps on the other hand are known as pulling motions or exercises. Therefore, in the beginner level I designed a workout that involves two pushing motions together and two pulling motions together on separate days. Chest & Triceps are pushing exercises and usually done together by many people of all different levels. Back & Biceps are pulling exercises that are also performed by many people of all different levels. Like I said before and will say again, there is no wrong or right order to doing these exercises – you can mix-and-match or do what you think works best for you. Your body, however, needs constant change and in no way can get accustomed to same movements, motions, frequency and intensity. Boring workouts should never be a word used in your vocabulary for weight training.

<u>Workout #1 – Chest & Biceps</u> (this is known as a push/pull split routine)

Flat-Bench Barbell Presses - 4 sets of 12, 10, 8, 8 repetitions (increase the weight after every set and rest approximately 30 seconds)

Smith Machine Incline Presses – 4 sets of 12 repetitions (keep the same weight and see the sick pump you get from these sets)

Flat Dumbbells Fly's – 4 sets of 12, 12, 10, 10 repetitions (increase the weight and make sure that your form is on point)

Incline DB Fly's – 4 sets of 10 repetitions (keep the same weight and just focus on your contraction to ensure a good pump)

Alternate DB Curls – 4 sets of 15 repetitions (increase the weight after every set and rest only 30 seconds to ensure that burning sensation)

Preacher Curls (any grip you desire) – 4 sets of 12, 10, 8, 8 repetitions (increase the weight and make sure you go down to a complete range of motion)

Concentration Curls – 3 sets of 15, 12, 10 repetitions (make sure you increase the weight)

OR

Incline DB Presses – 4 sets of 12, 12, 10, 8 repetitions (increase the weight and make sure that your form is perfect – meaning that you lower the dumbbells to at least a 90 degree angle. This will make the upper part of your chest work harder)

Incline DB Fly's – 4 sets of 10 repetitions (keep a challenging weight)

Cable Crossovers – 4 sets of 15 repetitions (increase the weight a drop and make sure that you squeeze hard at the end of the movement. This makes the inner chest more defined and extremely striated).

Pec-Dec Fly's – 4 sets of 10 repetitions (increase the weight)

21's – you can use a barbell since working with dumbbells requires much more balance and strength (use an Olympic bar or a fixated barbell and do three sets of this exercise)

Dumbbell Curls – 3 sets of 15 repetitions (use both arms at the same time). You will really begin to feel a burn in both the biceps and forearms. If you also begin to feel it in the

deltoids then chances are the weight is heavy or you might be leaning slightly forward and shifting the weight to your shoulders.

Wide-Grip Cable Curls – 4 sets of 10, 10, 15, 15 repetitions (this is challenging because you are starting with a heavier weight and lower for the last two sets lowering the weight to an easier amount to make sure you are able to squeeze out 15 grueling repetitions. Wow this burns and yes you will begin to sweat and scream).

So these are only two different workouts for chest and biceps – both are challenging and require time, effort and focus. The repetitions are not high as in the beginner level but the weight is a bit more challenging and demanding. Do not rush these workouts and pay extra attention to your form. If you need to decrease the weight to get the required repetitions and sets then please do. There is no need to show off and complete these routines with half-ass form. The second chest workout that I listed is designed for those who want their upper chest (clavicle) to grow and look bigger. In regards to the bicep routine all I can say is good luck it is challenging and well it burns.

Workout #2 Legs

Leg Extensions – 2 sets of 20 repetitions at a light weight (warm-up)

Smith Machine Squats – 4 sets of 15 repetitions (if you can go heavier than do so, but I don't think you will)

Leg Presses – 4 sets of 12, 12, 10, 10 repetitions (this is a power movement so go heavy but be smart at the same time. High repetitions with heavier weight can be extremely challenging).

Leg Extensions – 4 sets of 15, 12, 10, 8 repetitions (this is no longer a warm-up so increase the weight after every set and make sure you are getting a full range of motion and a good contraction)

Leg Curls – 4 sets of 15 repetitions (keep the weight steady and make sure you can complete the sets with proper form)

OR

Alternate Lunges – 4 sets of 15 repetitions (use a barbell or a smith machine and this means that each leg is doing 15 repetitions so that at the end of this exercise each leg did 60 lunges)

Squats (barbell or smith machine) – 4 sets of 12, 12, 10, 10 repetitions (increase the weight and watch your thighs increase in size)

Leg Extensions – 4 sets of 15 repetitions (increase the weight after every set)

Stiff-Legged Deadlifts (either a barbell or dumbbells) – 4 sets of 15 repetitions (increase the weight slightly)

Leg Curls – 3 sets of 12 repetitions (strict and tight)

These leg workouts are extremely challenging and need to be done all alone. Each routine should take you no longer than 40-45 minutes with appropriate resting time. You will sweat tremendously and even be out of breath at times so make sure you are drinking plenty of liquids and breathing effectively. The build up of lactic-acid in the leg muscles is like no other and boy will it burn. But, rather than quitting with the feeling of vomiting, stick it through and continue with the workout even if you have to decrease the weight, repetitions or sets. You will feel better when the workout is completed or right after you vomit. In addition, the reason I chose to do legs on workout #2 was because your upper body will be sore from the chest and bicep routine so it is a good way to give the upper body some rest.

<u>Workout #3 Back & Triceps</u> (this is also known as a push/pull split routine)

Pull-Up's – 3 sets of 12 repetitions (any grip you desire and if that is too hard for you, then most gyms have a gravitron unit. This is a machine that gives you some help in doing a pull-up by supporting some or most of your weight. Your knees are rested on a platform that will help you contract and complete the movement. Once you develop some strength to lift your own full body weight then this unit is no longer needed.

Wide-Grip Lat Pull downs – 4 sets of 15, 15, 10, 10 repetitions (increase the weight after every set and make sure to squeeze in your shoulder blades)

One-Arm DB Rows – 3 sets of 12 repetitions (nice and strict and keep the weight constant)

Cable Rows (close-grip) – 4 sets of 12, 10, 8, 8 repetitions (increase the weight after every set and make sure your back is straight and that you are getting your full range of motion)

Rope Pressdowns – 4 sets of 15, 12, 10, 8 repetitions (increase the weight and make sure that your elbows are at your side at all times)

Skull-Crushers – 3 sets of 12 repetitions (increase the weight)

Close-grip Pressdowns – 4 sets of 15 repetitions (increase the weight and hold at the bottom of the movement for a second)

Dips (either weighted on two benches or a dip station) – 3 sets of 12 repetitions (make sure to lock at the end of the movement)

OR

One-Arm DB Rows – 4 sets of 12 repetitions (increase the weight)

Wide-Grip Lat Pulldowns – 4 sets of 12, 12, 10, 10 repetitions

Close-Grip Lat Pulldowns – 4 sets of 15 repetitions (use correct form and make sure that the contraction is felt)

Reverse Underhand Grip – 4 sets of 10, 10, 8, 8 repetitions (go heavy on this motion and make sure you feel it in your back and biceps as well)

Hyperextensions – 3 sets of 20 repetitions

Overhead DB Extension – 4 sets of 12 repetitions (increase the weight slightly)

V-Bar Pressdowns – 4 sets of 10, 10, 10, 20 repetitions (increase the weight after every set and for the fourth set lower the weight and make sure that you are able to get 20 repetitions. This allows for a great pump and a huge amount of blood in the triceps).

Dumbbell Kickbacks – 4 sets of 12 repetitions (same weight and make sure that your elbow is by your side and not flared out)

These two different workouts for these muscle groups are very challenging and really great for results. They are designed in a way that allows the body to work at its hardest so that results can easily be seen. Try to pace yourself accordingly so that your workouts do not last more than 45 minutes. These workouts will also keep your heart rate up and allow you to develop a good amount of endurance.

Workout #4 – Shoulders & Trap's (remember I said you can also mix-and-match exercises and order of workouts to better fit your schedule and demands).

DB Shoulder Presses – 4 sets of 20, 15, 12, 10 repetitions (increase the weight after your first warm-up set and see how your shoulders begin to burn)

DB Lateral Raises – 4 sets of 15 repetitions – strict form and make sure you don't use any momentum. You can perform this exercise either seated or standing. Just make sure it is strict and correct.

Frontal Raises – 4 sets of 12, 10, 10, 10 repetitions (increase the weight and make sure your back is straight and knees slightly bent. If you are rocking and using your knees then lean up against a wall to ensure proper form).

Upright Rows (Barbell or Smith Machine or Cable station using a straight bar) – 4 sets of 15, 15, 8, 8 repetitions (increase the weight and make sure your form is accurate)

DB Shrugs – 4 sets of 12 repetitions (definitely increase the weight on this exercise and try to make your traps touch your ear. This is not really possible but if you try you will be bound in getting a full range of motion with a super contraction. While doing these shrugs make sure to never round your shoulders and use momentum by bending your knees up and down. Keep a straight posture and hold the dumbbells by your sides with a slight bend in the elbows.

OR

Military Presses (Barbell or Smith Machine) – 4 sets of 12, 10, 8, 6 – increase the weight and make sure your using the right amount of weight to get the following repetitions

Arnold Presses – 4 sets of 15 repetitions (use a steady and manageable weight and these repetitions will begin to burn)

Lateral Raises – 4 sets of 12 repetitions (this is a perfect routine to follow-up Arnold Presses with)

Reverse-Pec-Dec Fly's – 3 sets of 15, 12, 10 repetitions (increase the weight)

Smith Machine Shrugs – 4 sets of 15 repetitions (increase the weight and keep perfect form and posture)

Both of these shoulders routines are challenging and are absolutely perfect for attacking all the three heads of the deltoids. The first routine is mostly all dumbbells and as you figured out by now I love dumbbells. The second routine is a good combination of free weights and dumbbells. You can really feel your shoulders working with both these routines and once again feel free to mix around exercises and format to better suit your needs.

So now that we covered the intermediate level exercises and routines we can go into the advanced levels. The basic routines gave you the essential exercises, sets and repetitions needed to familiarize yourself with how the body works. It is the basis for almost every body type and desired goal. You are gaining a bit of strength, an increase in your endurance levels and the ability to understand proper form and coordination. As you became familiarized with many exercises and movements you developed an understanding – a sound knowledge of what your abilities and potentials are. The intermediate level challenged you and really made you anxious, or even, curious, as to what else your body can endure. You were pounded with heavier weights, compound exercises, numerous sets and absolutely a vigorous schedule. Yet you stuck it through and some of you even breezed through these workouts and skipped right into the advanced routines – round of applause to you. Fitness done one way, the right way, is what I preach and what I practice. I mentioned so many times as to how incorrect or inconsistent people work out. This book prepares you for all the levels by listing exercises along with pictures and explanations and also serves as a motivational tool for those who need or needed that extra push. Inspiration is a good word to describe what fitness is to me and for so many others and is my main reason for writing this book – to inspire the uninspired.

Part III – Advanced Routines, Exercises and Programs (these routines were dug up from the archives and are strenuous, demanding and, oh yea, HARD).

So now that we came across the advanced routines all I can say is that everything we spoke about up till now is going to be used - all those principles and methods, different exercises, angles and degrees. Your body will begin to undergo substantial changes. Many will become bigger, leaner, stronger, extremely defined and muscular. While not everybody will see immediate results, I guarantee that all will feel better, sleep better and even look better. A sense of pride and accomplishment become imminent and soon you will have the confidence and the ability to reach your desired goals, needs and wants. So the advanced routines will require all that was just mentioned so why not approach these routines with the feeling of determination – either you conquer, or become conquered. I will list a few routines for different muscles and will label them as workouts #1, #2, etc... The typical routines are for at least 4 or 5 days with a day in between for rest and recovery. Once again feel free to pick whichever workout routines adhere to you and your busy schedule.

So this workout was designed by me as a means to get bigger before I competed again. It was a 12 week program (3 months) and absolutely perfect for gaining muscle mass.

12-week growth program

Workout #1 – Chest/Traps/Biceps/Abdominals – seems like way too much to do in an hour but I was able to manage and if you pace yourself accordingly so can you. I usually always start Mondays off with chest because it gives me the pump and power needed to sustain my workouts for the week.

Incline DB Presses – 5 sets of 15, 12, 10, 8, 8 repetitions (increase the weight and rest only 30 seconds before you go again)

Incline Smith Machine Presses – 4 sets of 12, 12, 10, 8 repetitions (increase the weight and make sure that you lower the bar almost ½ inch to your chest. Once again rest 30 seconds before you begin your next set. I guarantee that by this point you are pumped beyond belief and even developed a sweat).

Incline Fly's – 3 sets of 10 repetitions (use a moderate weight that is challenging)

Cable Crossovers – 3 sets of 15 repetitions (increase the weight and make sure you squeeze hard at the end of the movement)

DB Shrugs – 4 sets of 15, 12, 10, 8 repetitions (increase the weight and keep strict form)

Smith Machine Shrugs – 4 sets of 12 repetitions (increase the weight and use either an overhand grip or one hand under the bar grip)

Preacher Curls (close-grip) – 4 sets of 12, 12, 10, 8 repetitions (increase the weight and make sure your elbows are on the pad and close together)

Preacher Curls (wide-grip) – 4 sets of 12, 12, 10, 8 repetitions (same as above)

Concentration Curls – 3 sets of 12 repetitions (use a constant weight and make sure your form is perfect)

Hammer Curls – 1 set to failure (failure means till you are extremely exhausted and can't even do one forced repetition)

<u>Workout #2 – Back & Deltoids</u> – this becomes challenging because you might still either be sore from the previous bicep routine or just fatigued

Wide-Grip Lat Pull downs – 6 sets of 15, 15, 12, 12, 10, 10 repetitions (increase the weight after every set and maintain proper form throughout)

Wide-Grip Pull-Up's – 4 sets of 12 repetitions (if challenging for you then try to reach a total of 25 repetitions for as long as it takes. I once did 52 pull-up's in two sets with a 30 second rest. My first set consisted of 29 repetitions and my second set was followed by 23 repetitions. I love pull-up's and always up for a challenge when it comes to any form of pull-up. They are a true sense of strength and an excellent exercise.

One-Arm DB Rows – 3 sets of 10 repetitions (keep a heavy weight)

Close-grip Lat Pull downs – 3 sets of 12 repetitions (use a normal weight that is fair so that this exercise can function as your cool down)

Frontal Dumbbell Raises – 4 sets of 12 repetitions (increase the weight and make sure that your elbows are only slightly bent)

Bent-Over Lateral Raises either seated or standing – 4 sets of 12, 12, 10, 10 repetitions (increase the weight)

Dumbbell Presses – 4 sets of 10, 10, 8, 6 then right back to 15 repetitions (increase the weight for all four sets and after the 4th set is completed for 6 reps lower the weight to about 50% less and immediately perform 15 repetitions. This is known as a drop-set, remember?)

Lateral DB Raises – 3 sets of 15 repetitions (keep the same weight – this is also a good way to burn out and totally fatigue the shoulders.)

This back and deltoid routine is complicated to complete because of the power exercises and both the amount of repetitions required and the increase in weight. However, they are not as hard as some of the workouts I experienced over the years. You are more than experienced and educated up to this point so go ahead and tackle these workouts. Caution, this back and deltoid routine will really get you going and even give you the feeling that you can carry the weight of the world on your back and shoulders.

<u>Workout #3 – Quadriceps/Hamstrings/Calves/Triceps</u> (In previous chapters I mentioned that when doing legs you should dedicate a day for them all alone. The idea stills stays the same except for the fact that you will be doing legs with a small muscle group. The triceps are not a major muscle group where they need to be worked out all alone so doing them after legs should be just fine. There won't be a sudden change in blood pressure or blood and oxygen flow since the triceps are a small muscle group. From past experiences I noticed that whenever I did legs with a larger muscle group (chest, back or shoulders) I began to almost always get nauseas and light-headed or dizzy. But, while doing legs and then triceps I noticed no sudden changes and was able to complete both body parts in harmony and in a timely fashion).

Leg Extensions – 4 sets of 15 repetitions (increase the weight after every set and make sure you are getting that full contraction)

Smith Machine Squats – 4 sets of 25 repetitions (use a light weight and make sure that each rep is done correctly and explosive. I must tell you, however, that 100 repetitions will absolutely burn the quadriceps/thighs).

Smith Machine Lunges – 4 sets of 15 repetitions (be sure that you have a good range of motion and that your back is straight with your knee about ½ inch off the floor. If you have knee issues then make sure your range of motion suits your ability and relieves pressure off the knees.

Leg Extensions – 4 sets of 15, 15, 12, 10 repetitions (increase the weight and feel the burn occurring almost immediately).

Leg Curls – 4 sets of 15, 15, 12, 12 repetitions (increase the weight)

Calves – try to design a workout on your own. Remember, you need to blast them in order for you to see results. So get creative and challenge this muscle to its ultimate maximum potential.

Skull-Crushers – 4 sets of 10, 10, 12, 15 repetitions (start with a heavy weight and decrease after the second and third sets)

Rope Pressdowns – 4 sets of 15 repetitions (increase the weight if you can)

Bench Dips – 4 sets of 15 repetitions (you can use weight if you are training with a partner)

Kickbacks using a Dumbbell – 1 set of 15 repetitions (use an easy weight that allows for proper and strict form)

If you read all the exercises and routines for the advanced level you might see that only three workouts were listed. At first glance you might think that it's not any harder than the intermediate levels but you are wrong. These three workouts require much more strength and time than you can imagine. They are strenuous and the reason I listed only three workouts is because a good amount of time is needed for recuperation and adequate rest. If you think this is not challenging then try to hit each body part twice in a week and see how sore and tired you become.

When I first opened my gym in 2007 I had a fifty-two year-old male client come into my place and ask me if he was able to get real lean and defined abdominals. My direct reply to him was I don't see why not – he had previous workout experiences and was in fairly decent shape so I began to examine his workout routines and see where we can make some alterations. He wanted to be challenged and gain a bit of muscle as well. Now gaining muscle and getting lean at the same time is almost nearly impossible but I have seen it done before. I really wanted to put him through some intense and vigorous workouts that would make him feel sick. I handed him a program and told him that he will need enough energy and motivation to get through this workout at 5:30 AM. Early workouts like this are extremely challenging considering your body is just waking up and majority of people I know don't usually have an appetite at this time of hour. The program I am about to list was strictly designed for him and was thoroughly reviewed by all of my trainers, a professional bodybuilder, as well as a close weight training partner of mine. So if you think the other three advanced workouts were easy then good luck with this one.

Day #1 (Monday) – Chest & Back

(1) Incline DB Presses Superset with Bent-Over Barbell Rows

(5 sets of 6, 8, 10, 12, and 15 – start off with a heavy weight and as the repetitions get higher begin to decrease the weight; unless you can find the strength to use the same weight)

(2) Flat barbell Presses Superset with One-Arm DB Rows

(5 sets of 6, 8, 10, 12, 15 – same sequence and order as the first exercise)

(3) Incline DB Fly's Superset with Wide-Grip Lat Pulldowns

(5 sets of 6, 8, 10, 12, 15 – same as all the rest)

(4) Cable Crossovers Superset with Close-Grip pull-Up's Superset with Hyperextensions – this is known as a tri-set or a Giant set. Three continuous exercises back-to-back-to-back.

(5 Sets of 10, 10, 12, 12, 15 – only exception with this is that hyperextensions can be performed for more than the required amount if possible)

Day #2 (Tuesday) – Shoulders/Traps & Triceps

DB Shoulder Presses Superset with Lateral DB Raises

(4 sets of 6, 8, 10, 12 – start with a challenging weight and decrease the weight by the 2nd or 3rd set, unless you can keep the same weight)

Front DB Raises Superset with Upright Rows

(4 sets of 6, 8, 10, 15 – same routine as the first exercise)

Arnold Presses Superset with Bent-Over DB Lateral Raises or Reverse Pec-Dec Fly's

(4 sets of 12, 10, 8, 6 – these two exercises are done a bit differently than the previous two because you start off with a light weight and work your way up to a heavier weight with less repetitions)

DB Shrugs – **5 sets of 12, 12, 12, 8, 8 – use a moderate weight for the first three sets then increase the weight and decrease your repetitions**

Overhead DB Extension Superset with Rope Pressdowns

(4 sets of 10, 10, 15, 15 repetitions – try to maintain the same weight if possible but if you need to drop weight that is fine too)

V-Bar or Straight Bar Pressdowns Superset with Kickbacks

(4 sets of 10 repetitions using the same weight and maintaining strict form throughout)

Dips (either using a bench or a dip station) Superset with DB Skull Crushers

(4 sets of 12 repetitions – this becomes a great routine for cooling down since your repetitions are high and most probably your using a comfortable weight. In addition I am quite sure that the lactic acid building up in your triceps will cause immediate burning sensations)

Day #3 (Wednesday) – Legs/Calves/Abdominals

Leg Extensions w/ a one-second hold at the top

(5 sets of 10, 10, 12, 15, 20 – start with a fairly challenging weight and as the repetitions get higher you can start decreasing the weight, unless you can do that many repetitions with the same weight and 30 second rest in between each set)

Squats Superset with Leg Press (this can be real challenging and requires good breathing skills so that way you won't end up exhausted and struggling to catch your breath)

(4 sets of 15, 15, 10, 10 repetitions – start with a weight that you think is manageable on both exercises and make sure that the superset is done without any rest. You squat for the required repetitions and walk on over to the leg press machine and do the same. This will totally blow up your thighs and a massive amount of blood will be in that area – that is what creates the pump)

Lunges (either with Dumbbells or Barbell or Smith Machine) Superset with Leg Curls

(4 sets of 15 repetitions - using the same weight though out all four sets. If you are strong and have both the endurance and power then increase the weight and maintain 15 repetitions)

Standing Calf Raises Superset with seated Calf raises

(5 sets of 15, 15, 15, 20, 25 repetitions – once again the weight disparity is totally up to you and how comfortable you feel)

Abdominals – at least 10-12 minutes of intense routines (you have plenty of exercises to work with)

Day #4 (Friday) – Chest & Biceps

Incline Barbell Presses (place the bench on 2nd level)

(4 sets of 10, 10, 10 ,10 repetitions – keep the same weight and rest just about 20 seconds and you will start to feel the burn in your shoulders, upper chest and triceps)

Incline Fly's Superset with Flat Fly's

(4 sets of 6, 8, 10, 12 – start heavy and work your way down on the dumbbell rack)

Pullovers Superset with Decline DB Presses

(4 sets of 10, 12, 15, 20 repetitions – this is a good routine for both the lower part of the chest as well as the entire rib cage and inner chest. If you have to decrease the weight after each set then by all means do)

Barbell Curls Superset with Alternate DB Curls

(4 sets of 12, 12, 10, 8 repetitions – you must rest 30 seconds and no more and continue using strict form without any rocking or jerking movements. Try to maintain the same weight but if you must then go ahead and lower the weight)

Preacher Curls (close-Grip) Superset with Wide-Grip cable Curls

(4 sets of 12, 10, 8, 6 repetitions – start light then go heavy)

Hammer Curls

(3 sets of 15 repetitions using a moderately light weight)

<u>Day #5 – pick any one or two body parts that you either think need work on or just feel like you didn't get a good enough workout on the previous days.</u>

So after a month of sticking to this routine my client came by my gym and boy did he look absolutely good. Like I said before he was in great shape to begin with but now he was a bit leaner and defined and was also able to maintain the same weight. He looked more muscular and thick while still being extremely shredded and lean. I guess this routine worked for him and I think it can work for so many others. The 5 day workout routine was vigorous and required lots of stamina and a true commitment to sticking it through. It is a heavy workload with both heavy weights for muscle mass and then light weights with crazy amounts of repetitions for that shredded look. The aforementioned workouts require dedication, time, patience and an overall passion for reaching your potential. Every body part should be treated equally and given the same amount of attention and rest to guarantee proper results. Treat every one of your workouts like it's your last. Before I completely end this segment, I feel obligated to leave you guys with one more routine that happens to be my favorite routine. Once again feel free to coordinate the days and times to your schedule. I consider this routine to be a competition exercise program and I learnt this particular workout from Arnold Schwarzenegger's Encyclopedia as well as my old time bodybuilder training partner, mentor and close friend.

<u>Day #1 – Chest & Back & Abdominals</u>

Bench Presses Superset with Wide-Grip pull-Up's (5 sets of 10 repetitions – increase the weight on the Bench Presses and maintain a 30 second rest in between each set)

Incline Dumbbell Presses Superset with Close-Grip Pull-Up's (4 sets of 10 repetitions – once again increase the weight on the Incline DB Presses and rest 30 seconds in between sets)

Incline DB Fly's Superset with T-Bar Rows (4 sets of 10 repetitions – increase the weight, if possible, for both exercises and take 30 second rests in between sets)

Cable Crossovers Superset with Wide-Grip Lat Pulldowns (4 sets of 10 repetitions – increase the weight for both exercises and rest 30 seconds in between sets)

Abdominals

Seated Leg Tucks (4 sets of 25 repetitions with only a 10 or 15 second rest)

Crunches (4 sets of 25 repetitions with only a 10 or 15 second rest and make sure that you squeeze hard and get a good contraction)

Hanging Leg raises (4 sets of 25 repetitions with no momentum or swinging motions)

Day #2 – Shoulders & Biceps & Triceps

Barbell Presses Superset with DB lateral Raises (4 sets of 10 repetitions – increase the weight if you can and maintain strict form while only resting for 30 seconds in between sets)

Arnold Presses Superset with Bent-Over DB Laterals (4 sets of 10 repetitions – increase the weight, if possible, and make sure you complete the required amount of repetitions)

Upright Rows (barbell or smith machine) Superset with DB Frontal Raises (4 sets of 10 repetitions – increase the weight and maintain strict form throughout)

Arms (Biceps & Triceps)

Barbell Curls (shoulder-width grip) Superset with Skull Crushers (4 sets of 10 repetitions – increase the weight if you can and take no rest in between the actual superset. Once you complete a set then rest for 30 seconds – this will really begin to burn and give you a good pump)

Alternate DB Curls (standing or seated) Superset with Rope Pressdowns (4 sets of 10 repetitions – increase the weight a drop and make sure your elbows are at your side the whole time for both exercises)

Concentration Curls Superset with Dips [weighted bench dips or on a dip station] (4 sets of 10 repetitions – keep the weight constant unless you are doing weighted bench dips. If so then go ahead and have your partner put some plates on you and to make things interesting begin to drop set)

Day #3 – Legs & Calves & Abdominals

Leg Extensions (1 set of 25 repetitions – light weight and only used for a warm-up)

Barbell Squats (4 sets of 10 repetitions – try increasing the weight and resting 30 seconds in between sets)

Lunges - holding DB's by your side(4 sets of 10 repetitions on each leg – maintain good form and make sure your back is straight and your knees never go past your feet/toes)

Leg Presses (4 sets of 10 repetitions – increase the weight and if you want you can begin to change foot positioning to feel the difference in the inner and outer thighs)

Leg Extensions Superset with Stiff-Legged Deadlifts [DB or Barbell] (4 sets of 10 repetitions – increase the weight and rest 30 seconds between each set. Your thighs should be on fire already but if not they will be now)

Calves

Standing calf Raises Superset with Seated Calf Raises (4 sets of 25 repetitions – increase the weight and rest 30 seconds in between each set)

Donkey Calf Raises (4 sets of 10 repetitions – increase the weight)

Abdominals

Crunches on the floor (4 sets of 50 repetitions)

Machine Crunches (4 sets of 25 repetitions)

Day #4 – Rest and Recovery (make sure you get enough sleep and consumption of protein and good carbohydrates)

Day # 5 – Repeat of Day #1

Day #6 – Repeat of Day #2

Day #7 – Repeat of Day #3

Ok so this is an advanced workout, obviously, and entails you to work out 6 days with one rest day to fully recuperate. The routines are compound and involve much of my favorites: 30 second rests and supersetting two different body parts. This also allows you to work each and every body part twice a week with direct and strenuous movements. I must warn you now that this routine is extremely challenging and requires more attention than you can imagine. It was also the routine that began to set me back – overtraining was clearly forthcoming and hit me like a ton of bricks. Don't fall into my traps and allow yourself plenty of time to recover and time to just break away once you feel any strange feelings. I ignored these signs and never listened to my body. Thus, I suffered deeply with depression, loss of stamina and an overall desire to quit. That is what overtraining can do and it sneaks up on you so listen to your body and respond immediately.

Part IV – synopsis of the three training levels

So now that we have elaborated on the beginner, intermediate and advanced levels we need to review a few more important issues. One might ask when and where do you actually do abdominals; oblique's, forearms and calves? Well the answer is simple – I do them every other day. I did not go into specifics with exercises for those body parts because I like every individual to pick their own exercises and routines they feel comfortable with. Remember, these body parts should be trained with accuracy and treated like any other muscle group. Again, the answers for these questions all depend on your goals, time constraints and schedule. These smaller muscles are just as important and really need to be trained properly to complement your overall physique. Another question you might be pondering is how often should I do

Cardio/Aerobic exercises or should I do it before or after my weight training workouts? Again, the answer depends on your goals. All three levels of weight training routines listed in a way are a form of aerobic exercises. The fact that you are going through your workouts within 45 minutes and 30 second rest in between sets and exercises allows for an increased heart rate and heavy breathing. It will help you drastically in working on your endurance levels but that's about it. However, in no ways are these workouts considered anaerobic (without air) because once again you are only resting a minimal amount of seconds and moving at a quick pace.

Aerobic exercise is defined as any activities associated with the use of oxygen by the muscles. Many experts, bodybuilders, and sports professionals recommend that at least 30 minutes a day of physical activity is needed, whether in the form of cardio machines, aerobic classes or walking/jogging outdoors. I do some type of aerobic training for at least 20-30 minutes three to four days a week. Depending on your schedule and needs, doing cardio becomes more a matter of personal preference and a good way to strengthen your heart, lungs and circulatory system. Knowing and understanding your body type, goals and agendas are crucial for determining how to format your cardio routines. For example, individuals who are ectomorphic (slow gainers) and are slender with issues gaining weight should probably not do that much cardio since they don't have much energy and body fat to burn. When I was first starting to work out my main objective was to gain both weight and some muscle mass so I limited my cardio sessions to twice a week for approximately 30 minutes. Those trying to lose some body fat and shed a few extra pounds can benefit from more frequent cardio and aerobic sessions. Maybe work yourself up to 45 minutes or an hour, 4 or 5 days a week. Like with any other program or routine, you must first get acclimated to certain motions, movements and breathing patterns. Start out slowly and give your body a chance to get used to it, especially while doing cardio. First you need understanding so that your progress can be easily reached without any interruptions, concerns or injuries. Believe me, running on a treadmill is not as easy as one might think it is. It requires intensity, commitment and understanding of what both the machine is capable of doing and your body is capable of performing. Doing cardiovascular exercises can be done on either the same day as your weight training routines or if your schedule allows on different days. So the answers are always depending on your schedule and your needs, do what suits you best.

Part V – Cardiac Arrest – rundown of some Cardio Machines

We all see these huge fancy looking machines in every gym. They are those big futuristic looking pieces of machines and some might even wonder if they can take us to the moon. No they don't yet have the capabilities of leaving the ground but you never know with the current advancements in the fitness industry. A cardiovascular exercise, or cardio for short, is a great way to help burn calories, lose weight, become more active, build endurance and even test coordination. I mean how many people do you know can walk on a treadmill while chewing gum, talking on the phone and watching television? The answer is almost everyone (lol). Cardio has been proven to make our hearts stronger, help reduce the risk of heart attack, high cholesterol, high blood pressure and diabetes. In addition it makes you feel good while reducing your stress levels dramatically. I have made numerous references to cardio training as well as aerobic training and will now list a few good pieces of cardio equipment.

Manufactures have produced cardio equipment in either a commercial grade or a residential grade to better enhance their consumers choices, possibilities and preferences. These pieces of equipment also come in different types of sizes, customizations and dimensions. Most cardio machines can stimulate activities, such as hiking, walking, climbing, running, peak and interval training amongst others. They can be used for those who are advanced or even those who are beginners. Sit back relax and try to determine which piece of equipment suits you best.

Treadmill – this piece of equipment is very common and most commercial gyms have dozens of them. Life Fitness produces a nice line of treadmills with all different specifications. You can get a basic treadmill that reads your heart rate and has some type of shock absorption or you can step up to one that has an ipod dock, small television screen in the middle of the unit and even has workouts programmed for you. In addition they can gather information and give you feedback about your cardio session. It can tell you the amount of calories burned, distance traveled, speed and etc. They all range in prices and the more specs you need the more you will have to shell out. Treadmills are great machines because they can suit all shapes of people and sizes and happens to be the most popular of the cardiovascular equipment categories. Walking, jogging, running and climbing are among the most prevalent forms of exercise worldwide. There are so many debates as to which cardio machine works best. Like anything else we have discussed so far you simply need to choose the machine which you think works best for you. If you have knees problems or back injuries be sure to ask for advice or even seek out answers on your own. Life Fitness, PreCor, Nordic Track and many other manufacturers carry plenty of cardio equipment and are highly recognizable and reputable. I enjoy using the treadmill and feel it works great for me. However, many of my clients that have knee issues or bad posture I try to avoid using the treadmill. It places a great deal of stress and impact on the knees and most often you get people holding on to the bars and leaning down on it. Posture, balance, coordination and stability are key components for good results on this machine. I hate when my clients use the treadmill and complain of severe knee and lower back pains. So as a trainer I improvise and place them on another piece of cardio equipment like the stationary bike.

Stationary Bike – this is probably the second most popular cardiovascular machine. Stationary bikes are the least expensive type of equipment and take up less space than treadmills and ellipticals. These bikes for me act as a great tool to warm up my clients as well as cool them down after a workout session. They are low on impacting the knees and serve well for most of your needs. Overall a pretty useful piece of equipment, even if it turns out to be a spot to place your clothes on or become a storage space.

Elliptical or Cross-Training Machines – these machines are fairly new and are being changed and improved almost constantly. They usually resemble an egg-shape and have really big looking pedals. All these elliptical machines from every company work the muscles of the lower and upper body, with forward and backward pedal motions to minimize impact to ankles, knees, hips and lower back. These X-trainers (ellipticals) also come with heart rate reading capability, distance traveled, speed (RPM), time and calories burned. In addition, the majority of them have at least 16 levels of resistance to better enhance your workouts and your goals. I find these machines to be incredibly challenging and demanding. After a 12 minute use on level 2 with the speed at 6.0 I come off this machine at a high heart rate, sweaty body and physically fatigued. Again, there is no clear cut answer as to which machine is better – it is largely a matter of exercisers' personal preferences.

Stair Climbers – when I first started working out stair climbers were a dime a dozen and were extremely popular. I would see men, women, bodybuilders and athletes using these machines with puddles of sweat by their feet. It is a challenging machine and as you get more inclined to its motions and resistance it tends to get harder and harder. However, today most gyms only carry a small amount of these star climbers because of the impact it has on your knees and lower back. Many manufacturers endured many lawsuits and had no choice but to totally improve these machines. They are now real futuristic looking and actually less intimidating. They have much more shock absorbers and even a smoother appeal to both its movements and resistance. Life Fitness, my absolute favorite, produces a few nice versions of this machine and I enjoy using them. I really feel this machine the most out of all the others mentioned. I sweat tremendously and really feel differences in my legs and calves. So I guess why not give this machine a try since you have nothing else to lose except weight.

I recommend that once you begin doing cardio you purchase a heart rate monitor. The brand POLAR makes a telemetry band that goes around your chest to get the most accurate heart rate reading. It is affordable and works perfect with every cardio machine and even great for weight training since the band comes with a digital watch displaying your heart rate. The chest strap sends your heart rate readings to a special wrist watch which translates the information into numbers and easy for you to comprehend. Once you learn what your target heart is or should be these numbers on the watch will start to make more sense. According to the topendsports.com website normal resting heart rates should be anywhere from 40 to 100 beats per minute. Ideally you want it to be between 60-90 beats per minute, with the average resting heart rate for a man being 70 beats per minute, and for a woman 75 beats per minute. During exercise, your heart rate will depend on the intensity, frequency, age and your fitness level(s). While performing any type of exercise, especially cardio, you want your maximum heart rate to be recorded. Your maximum is the highest number of heart beats per minute while exercising vigorously. This 220 minus your age formula is not always accurate but does a good job coming close to averaging your maximum heart rate. The results are usually averaged and used for training levels, guides, diagrams and charts. You will always see some type of chart on any piece of cardio equipment showing what the target heart rate should be for every age group. It is usually done by ACSM – American College of Sports Medicine and usually changes yearly or so with regards to obesity, diabetes, heart attacks and other medical factors. After all we are the nation's rising health concern and obesity is among so many of us. Below is an example of what these charts look like and remember they are not always 100% accurate.

AGE	Max HR
10	210
11	209
12	208
13	207
14	206
15	205
16	204
17	203
18	202
19	201
20	200
21	199
22	198
23	197
24	196
25	195
26	194
27	193
28	192
29	191
30	190
31	189
32	188
33	187
34	186
35	185
36	184
37	183
38	182
39	181
40	180
41	179
42	178

43	177
44	176
45	175
46	174
47	173
48	172
49	171
50	170
51	169
52	168
53	167
54	166
55	165
56	164
57	163
58	162
59	161
60	160
61	159
62	158
63	157
64	156
65	155
66	154
67	153
68	152
69	151
70	150
71	149
72	148
73	147
74	146
75	145
76	144

77	143
78	142
79	141

Part VI – Overtime Training (Overtraining)

With all the many routines, exercises and limited time to train, we sometimes find ourselves overworked, overwhelmed and overtrained. Every set, repetition, exercise and routine can begin to take a pounding on the body and its inner functions. We begin to go through stages of anxiety, problems falling asleep, memorizing certain things, loss of energy, depression and a few others. Overtraining is a condition you go through from too much exercise over too much time. Certain mechanisms in the body that supply you with energy and which allow your body to recuperate and function become depressed or even shut down. It is a chronic state in which your body just can't perform anymore no matter how hard you try or push – your body shuts down and doesn't cooperate anymore at all. This is a common issue that many people deal with all the time; except no one knows how to deal with it and what they need to do. Your main response to overtraining should come in the form of rest. Not a day or two but maybe weeks. That doesn't mean you have to be in bed for that duration. Rather it means that your body is asking for a certain amount of time before you go back to working out and you must do exactly as your body says. I encountered all of the above characteristics of overtraining and I do not wish them upon anyone. It was so peculiar to know that at one time you feel like a champion, a million dollars, while on another day you are depressed, saddened and have absolutely no drive or energy for working out. The body is an extremely phenomenal creation and can take you to places you never imagined to go physically. However, do not overlook the fact that it requires rest and adequate time for recovery. This overtraining syndrome is fairly common and to avoid any levels of it just to be sure to follow these small steps and remember that "less is sometimes more."

- Make sure you get enough rest and adequate recovery time

- Make sure you are consuming enough nutrients, vitamins and minerals

- Do not go overboard on weight training, cardiovascular training or any other form of exercise

- Listen to your body and treat it right and in return it will treat you better

- Drink plenty of liquids

- Consume PROTEIN

Chapter 11
Tell Me the Truth – Some Issues
Need to Be Addressed

I love when clients and friends tell me that they are on a diet and doing cardio for weight loss. I always get a kick out of this one – I mean yes dieting is great and cardio is perfect for the heart and breathing. But, where does the weight loss come from? What happens to that fat and how do we make it tighter, firmer and muscular? I guess they didn't think those questions through. I have yet to see someone lose drastic weight from only doing cardio and dieting. We all know that dieting is about 90 percent of the battle for any effective weight training regiment and works great for weight loss and gaining weight as well. With only doing cardio chances are you will have much more energy and stamina within a few months, or weeks of starting regular aerobic activities. You will be able to last longer in most events requiring endurance but you might also feel fatigued or sore in the muscles quicker since you have been neglecting them. Perfect or peak conditioning requires absolute attention to every muscle group in your body. There has to be an order – an absolute proportion and placement to achieve overall perfection. You can't only work out the heart and forget about the legs. I mean while you're doing cardio are you noticing that your legs are the body parts that allow you to run, stride, glide and walk? So why not work them out as well so they can better aid you in the long run. If you're making an effort to lose weight and strengthen your heart then why not put an effort into working out your entire body from head-to-toe. No one said that you need to be a bodybuilder or a fitness model but it wouldn't hurt to have a natural and proportioned physique. In addition to all that was stated and on the issue of nutrition, weight loss depends on your eating habits, your metabolism and your overall genetic makeup. These factors along with your commitment to exercise (cardio and weight training) will speed the process and better aid you in the long run – trust me.

With adequate exercise, dieting, recuperation and knowledge, some are still curious about the performance of certain pills, protein powders and supplements. Many people I come across are constantly popping the latest "miracle pills" like candy as an effort to: burn fat, gain muscle, increase energy levels, get stronger, get more veins, increase sex drive, increase memory and coordination levels and so many others. We are always looking for the quick and easy fix and are willing to pay any price for it. These pills, powders and supplements are expensive and usually do not last forever. Meaning that every month or so you need to replenish your stock. You cling on to your "miracle goods" like a mother clings onto her new born baby. Some will see results while others will only wonder why they don't see any. Besides all the potentially harmful side effects people are still crowding GNC shops and other vitamin shops in a frenzy. No matter what pills or supplements you are ingesting or what diet you are following, just remember that experimenting is not a wise option and you should never treat your body like some type of research laboratory. Like I said before working out applies the same for these pills – what works for one person will not necessarily work for another. Everybody is different and unique in their own way and adapts to certain things differently. I have seen many friends and clients messing with the wrong pills or supplements and believe me it's never a nice sight for any eyes. Mood swings, hot flashes, dizziness, vomiting and even dehydration are some issues I dealt with regarding pills and supplements as a trainer and also as a competitor in natural bodybuilding shows. In this segment I will review some truths and myths about proper supplementation and fad diets. Just remember, in the game of fitness and healthy living there is absolutely no easy way out. It requires hard work and a true sense of commitment. So those gizmos, "miracle pills", diets and other such crap are all yesterday's news. The past is history, the future is a mystery and fitness is present and supersedes all.

Part I – Pill me in (which pills work and which pills do I use?)

The fitness and health industry has become one of the biggest money makers over the last few years. People are now becoming more aware of their bodies and what actually constitutes healthy living and a healthy lifestyle. Millions of dollars are spent annually on easy to get result items such as dietary supplements, protein powders and pills. You can't always believe what people say and what you read in magazines and see on television. However, we still become curious and even a bit misled to all the vast amounts of information and dabble here and there. Again we live in a society of lazy individuals who look for any easy way out so that the actual hard work can be undermined. What we don't know, however, about these supplements and pills are that most are not approved by the FDA (Food and Drug Administration) in the United States. The manufacturers don't have to prove that a supplement or pill is safe; the flip side is that the FDA has to prove whether or not the product is safe or dangerous before they can actually pull it off the shelves. I guess this works perfect for all those huge supplement manufacturers – they make these products with a catchy slogan and fancy models and sit back while the profits roll in. These big conglomerates that advertise these supplements in all fitness magazines most probably own the magazine and are able to advertise their products like crazy. Most of these supplements and pills in magazines promise to do a whole lot like "reduce body fat and increase lean muscle" and so much more. In most cases, maybe even all cases, these claims turn out to be frivolous and untrue. Before I continue, just remember to read all labels and do some research on the internet regarding the pills you want to start taking. Educating yourself on some of these issues will prevent you from making any accidental and harmful mistakes.

Fat-burning supplements and pills have been "hot" over the last few years. You can actually see many of these pills advertised everywhere you turn your head. The slogans are almost always similar and believable by so many people! Hey if I took these pills I can look like that model within no time is a common belief by so many naïve individuals. However, I can't really blame these people for thinking the way that they do. I mean after all we live in a capitalist society with only a desire to make money – and that is any way you can. These chiseled models along with some catchy slogans have paved way into mainstream America and become household figures and items. We try to imitate their diets, physiques, trends and, oh yea, take their pills all in the hopes of attaining lean muscle. I mentioned previous times that the best way to a lean and healthy life is: a nutritious diet, accompanied by physical exercise and appropriate rest and recuperation. Nevertheless, we American's believe that a shortcut is always tempting than the actual way and so therefore begin to spend crazy amounts of dollars on these so called "fat-burning" or "miracle" pills. Before discussing the many different fat-burning pills out there, we need to clearly understand that most people are using them to look great. I am a firm believer that feeling healthy supersedes looking great any time and comes with no harm or price. The main trouble spots for majority of people I know and trained are the abdominals, the oblique's (or as some call LOVE HANDLES) and the butt. Fact of the matter, you can actually get these areas of your body into great shape. It can also be done without any fat loss or fat-burning pills if you exercise regularly and follow good nutritional habits. But, who am I kidding – that is not like us and so therefore we will continue to use these fat burning pills as a means to dramatically speed up the process and maybe make it much easier.

Now before I begin listing a few fat-burning pills just remember that there are way too many of these pills for me to list and even know how each item works. I have never taken these pills but have many friends, gym partners and bodybuilders always giving me feedback regarding how they felt, looked and which items worked best for them. With these pills it's like going to Starbucks and ordering a venti Caramel Latte with Skim milk and a shot of whip cream. These pills come in all different shapes, sizes, and colors and can be catered to fit your expectations. The same way Starbucks can blend many coffees and drinks works the same exact way for these fat-burning pills and concoctions. However, in the back of every bottle of these pills you will find the following statement so be aware and take them at your own risk. *"These statements have not been evaluated by the Food and Drug Administration. This product is not intended to diagnose, treat, cure, or prevent any disease."*

Hydroxycut Hardcore is an extremely popular diet pill that is highly advertised on every workout magazine and particularly caters to male bodybuilders. This item has been around for a while now and used to be called just **Hydroxycut**. However, this products original formula contained Ephedra, a Chinese Herb used for helping with Hay fever and a common cold. Now banned by the FDA for quite a few years, **Hydroxycut** developed a new formula and renamed it **Hydroxycut hardcore.**

Xenadrine was once a famous fat-burning pill but because Ephedra was banned it lost a lot of its users. I don't recommend use of this pill because common side effects are: headaches, nervousness, cramps, increased sweating and increased heart rate, nausea and, at times, the feeling of being faint

Lipo-6 has been a great seller for the past few years now. I even think that it was rated the #1 fat burning pill for three years now. You see this being advertised in every bodybuilding magazine and I even think I saw it in men's Health once or twice. I don't have much information on this item except for the fact that it contains Synephrine, a common and highly used safe substitute to Ephedra.

Relacore is a diet pill that claims to help you lose weight by controlling your stress levels also known as cortisol levels. In my opinion I do not think that this fat-burning pill is good because the bottom line is that stress levels are not the only major factors contributing to weight problems.

Stacker 2 and Stacker 3 have been on the market for a good amount of time now. They also contained Ephedra until it was banned and people spoke highly of this product. A friend of mine once took this pill when there was Ephedra in it and absolutely loved the results. I asked him how did he feel and did he notice any changes and he replied "hell yeah I felt changes." When I asked him what they were he began listing me the following: increased blood pressure and heart rate, headaches, dizziness and at times light-headed, loss of appetite (I guess that can be both good and bad), nervousness, trouble falling asleep and at times extremely hyper active. Wow, what a price to pay for losing a few pounds. The new and improved **Stacker's** have most of what my friend experienced listed as possible side effects.

Fire Caps by CMI is pretty popular for giving someone that needed burst of energy. It acts as a thermogenic and allows your body to create mass amounts of heat (increased body temperature). This heat, supposedly, leads to weight loss and a crazy adrenaline rush. This product contains Ephedra and caffeine along with other ingredients to help you get through your intense workout. Have not heard much reviews of this product yet but I guess they are just as harmful as the ones I mentioned above.

Since I cannot write for days and days about each and every fat-burning pill on the market, I described and went over just a few. Just because something says that it will give you more energy and help you lose weight does not necessarily mean that it works. Think for a minute as to how many bottles of Ephedra, Caffeine or other stimulants you bought over the past few years? Most people I trained have spent more on these pills and supplements than on personal training sessions. A good amount of money and stupidity has been vested in these stimulants and some haven't been able to burn or shed an ounce of body fat. How pathetic.......... There are so many other ways to speed up your fat burning process and one of those is working out. Eating a healthy and properly balanced diet, along with exercise, rest and proper supplementation (vitamins) can further aid you in all your ventures. Don't waste your money on these fat-burning pills that don't work and have 101 harmful side effects. As mentioned so many times just because celebrities and athletes are endorsing specific brands of fat-burning pills and supplements don't mean that it will work for you. Endorsements are a money maker for these celebrities and I am quite sure that they will endorse whatever pays them the most and looks good on television and magazines.

Part II – tune in to PROTEIN

Should I be taking protein shakes before or after my workouts? Which protein powder works the best? How much protein should I consume a day? What foods are good to eat that are high in protein? Are RTD's (Ready-To-Drink) better than actual protein shakes? If you're working out then chances are you either heard these questions or have asked the same questions to others. Protein has always been a major issue for bodybuilders and with the recent trends in healthy living it is at the forefront of every diet. Most of us know that protein is needed by the body to build, repair and maintain muscle tissue and fiber. Protein is a substance that makes up your muscles, bones, cartilage, skin and all the enzymes in your body. Proteins in the body are broken down into amino acids – the building blocks. The body cannot use this protein you ingest without the help of all necessary amino acids. There are 22 amino acids present in proteins and of those 22, 13 are called nonessential amino acids while the remaining 9 are called essential amino acids. The human body cannot produce all of the necessary amino acids and can only rely on the foods you eat to supply the rest. Now who knew all that about protein? Now that we became a bit more educated and can actually understand what protein does, let's discuss some foods that contain protein before we move on to listing protein powders. As a bodybuilder and a trainer I always tried to consume about 1 to 2 grams of protein per pound. I was extremely conscious as to what foods were high in protein and easy to digest. The foods that I mostly ate for gaining weight and getting my daily hit of protein were:

Eggs (egg whites, yolks and in any fashion) – the best source of quality protein that is used by almost every bodybuilder, athlete, anyone and everyone.

Fish

Steak

Beef

Chicken

Cottage Cheese

Milk – including all milk products as well (cheese)

Soybeans, kidney beans, chick peas and other legumes

Protein bars & Protein Shakes

Now for the moment you have all been waiting for – Protein powders and shakes. Which are the best on the market and please give us a detailed evaluation of these powders? Ok so since you asked and I see you're curious, almost at the edge of your chair, I will review all the many protein powders I have tried over the last 10 years or so. Since eating a solid meal at times is tough and at times always impossible, protein shakes and ready to drink cans have become great selling items. All you need is either a blender or some type of shaker to put the powder in and add milk or water and you got yourself a high protein shake to fill you up and sustain you. While training for muscle or whatever it is you want to achieve it requires more than just hard work – it requires a good amount of protein. Considering the huge selection of powders at local GNC and other vitamin stores, one can easily become confused. Some protein powders promise one thing, while other promises another. They come in all different shapes, sizes, colors and prices. I was lost when I went to buy my first bottle of protein powder – I had absolutely no prior knowledge and all I did was listen to this small guy who said that this particular brand was the best seller. Of course I listened to him and gladly purchased what he gave me without even checking the price. I was 19 when I took my first shake and it was

Designer Whey Protein Powder in Chocolate flavor. To my demise, it was actually very tasty and easy to digest. However, back then not all protein powders in chocolate or vanilla were tasty – the exact opposite – they were chalky and extremely difficult to digest. But we all learn from experimenting and when I learned that I can use bananas, peanut butter, strawberries and other fruits to further enhance the taste and texture I was in protein heaven. So as the years went by and these manufacturers gained more recognition and success, better flavors and mixes were now put on shelves and selling out. The usual chocolate and vanilla were now overshadowed by flavors like chocolate malt, chocolate fudge, cookies and cream, creamy vanilla, alpine vanilla, strawberry, banana cream, and wow so many others. These manufacturers were getting smarter and smarter because they began to listen to consumers and science. They understand the human body and so therefore began to make powders that contain vital amino acids, creatine, vitamins and other great selling minerals and antioxidants. I absolutely love these shakes and tend to still have at least one a day after my workout or at times even on my days off. The taste is something I can never forget and the fact that I drink one a day is in no way a substitute for food. Food is the ultimate source of protein, vitamins and everything needed for the body to function. Civilization went through generations without a protein supplement and the same should be applied for us. If you need to use a shake or two for obvious reasons then go ahead, but remember that in no way should these shakes be treated as a substitute for real food. Below I will list a few Whey protein powders that I have tried, like and recommend.

Designer Whey Protein (French Vanilla) – this particular brand of protein powder is a safe and highly recognizable source. It has been around for a while now and they make it in a few different flavors but I enjoy the French vanilla with a scoop of peanut butter and a banana. In addition, at age 19 this powder seemed to be affordable as compared to many others. Good source of protein at a good price equals a smart and happy consumer.

EAS Myoplex Deluxe or Lite – depending on what you are using the protein for they make it lite (less calories) and deluxe (high in calories and used as a weight gainer). This happens to be a good product but overshadowed by many others.

Isopure (Alpine Vanilla or Dutch Chocolate) – a real good source of protein and a great seller. If you look at their website or any Isopure advertisement you will see the words pure and clean often. This company (which sells more than protein powders) developed protein so pure that it has absolutely no fat, no preservatives, no lactose, no calories and absolutely nothing to upset your stomach. They claim it to be 100% pure, 100% clean, 100% lite and 100% great tasting. It really is a well recognized company and their products are good and easy to digest. Only downfall is that their products are a bit pricy. I guess that's the price you have to pay for purity.

CytoSport Cyto Gainer (Vanilla) – this has been a top rated protein powder on many bodybuilding websites and happens to be one of my most recent favorites. I tell all my clients to use this powder and the majority of them end up loving the taste, texture and results. Great seller for all those hard-gainers out there. Try their many other different delicious flavors before you settle for the vanilla.

CytoSport Muscle Milk – wow these RTD's taste much better than a milkshake and are 100% more nutritional. This item can be purchased in protein powder or what I usually go for are the Ready to drink ones. Just pick one up, shake it well and enjoy. They make a good amount of flavors (chocolate milkshake, vanilla, cappuccino, banana crème, cake batter, mocha latte and so many others) and each one of them taste great. I am very pleased with their products and the protein blend is just as good as these RTD's.

Labrada Protein powder (lean body or PROV60 depending on your goals) – Lee Labrada is the founder, president and CEO of Labrada Nutrition. A former bodybuilder with many professional titles and a highly ranked bodybuilder, Mr. Labrada dedicated his time and effort to make American's more health conscious. He has over 20 years of experience in bodybuilding and nutrition and his products are just that good. He has been featured in many magazines and books as well as television (NBC, FOX, ABC, CBS, CNBC, ESPN and others) and stands by his products and his techniques to help shape American's. I enjoy his protein powders and most of his flavors too.

MuscleTech Nitro-Tech Protein (Vanilla & chocolate) – this product I have used plenty of times and had no problem digesting it and the taste was also pretty good. For those who don't know, MuscleTech is a huge company and all the major professional bodybuilders get signed to endorse their products. The advertisements are in every single health magazine (Flex, MuscleMag, Men's Health, Muscular Development and a few others) and bodybuilders like Dexter "Blade" Jackson, Jay Cutler, Branch Warren and so many others are highly used in all these ad's. Check out their website (www.MuscleTech.com) for a complete listing of their products and research.

Optimum 100% Whey Protein – this particular protein powder has won the protein powder of the year award for 2005, 2006 and 2007. The company is dedicated to raising the bar for the way protein powders are judged. They claim that their powder is pure and has more of what you want and none of what you don't need (fat, calories, carbohydrates, cholesterol, lactose and sugar). I believe that this powder is rated up there with the other pure blends and probably the most inexpensive.

BSN True-Mass (Vanilla Ice Cream or Chocolate Milk Shake) – this company produces those loud red bottles that you might see almost everywhere. Former Mr. Olympia, Ronnie Coleman, sponsors this company and they have had a great amount of success. Not a high rated protein blend but I used it for a few months while trying to gain some weight. Supposedly this mass gainer is designed for those people looking for additional calories as a means to gain muscle mass. It also contains a few key amino acids in its blend and some amino acids responsible for recovery and muscle growth. Overall a decent product and why not give it a try and judge for yourself.

Met-Rx – this company has been around for a while and I enjoy their products and all their advancements. I use to drink their protein powders as a meal replacement and boy did it fill me up. It was a great supplement to promote muscle growth. Their protein comes in already to use one single serving packet and tastes good. I enjoy the extreme chocolate flavor and on occasion drink their RTD's and eat their huge protein bars. I also love the fact that the World's Strongest Man Competition is sponsored by Met-Rx – my philosophy is that if their products are good for these strong men who lift cars then it is definitely good for a man of my size.

Okay so I listed my favorite 10 protein powers and hope that you pick one that suits you best. There are so many companies and products out there promising all different types of results. I tried many more blends then you can imagine and believe me not everyone was tasteful or digestible. I found myself in the toilet more often and at times with horrible stomach pains and cramps. Like anything else in this world, you learn from trial and error. I use these shakes as an addition to my meals. I never substitute food for shakes and I don't recommend that you do either. Food contains much more vitamins and minerals than many of these protein shakes and in no fashion should be replaced. In addition to these powders, the same manufactures developed protein bars as well. They act the same way a shake does except for the fact that it's in the form of a bar. Protein content is usually the same, give or take a few grams here and there and the taste is a bit different. These bars contain a bit more sodium, sugar, saturated fat and calories. Theses bars are a great snack for those who are either on the go or those who have some sort of sugar craving. Why not substitute that snickers bar with a nutritional protein bar instead. Trust me some of these protein bars can definitely put your taste buds into motion, as to compared with the bars from 8 years ago. The transformation of bars has undergone great advancements – they are now tastier, digestible, softer and chewable. I will list a few brands and flavors that I enjoy snacking on and hopefully you will agree with these choices:

Detour Bars made by Designer Whey in caramel peanut is my all time favorite. These bars are absolutely tasty and remind me of a snickers bar. It doesn't look like your typical protein bar and definitely doesn't taste like a protein bar either. I stock up on these bars and highly recommend them to my clients, friends and even some family members. The only downfalls about these bars are that they are high in sodium (400mg), high in calories (330 per bar) and carbohydrates (34 grams).

Promax Bars (cookies and cream) – just like the protein blend in their powders, this bar contains the same formula and is rich in protein. It is a great selling bar and at times compared to as a candy bar. It has a great texture and real easy to chew and enjoy. The only negative thing about this bar is that it's high in the sugar count (28 grams per bar) so don't overdose on these bars.

Met-Rx Big 100 Bars (Chocolate chip cookie dough or Chocolate chip graham cracker) – once again Met-Rx developed a high protein bar that's great tasting. The bars are fairly nutritional, low in fat and high in vitamins and antioxidants.

WSN Pure Protein Bar (chewy chocolate chip & chocolate deluxe) – these bars are affordable, extremely tasteful and packed with quality nutrients. I like the fact that these bars are delicious and low in calories, sugar and carbohydrates; another top favorite. In addition, these bars come in so many different flavors that I am quite sure you will find the ultimate flavor you have been waiting for.

Myoplex Lite or Deluxe Bars by EAS – these bars are a bit hard to digest and feel like you're chewing on a piece of rubber. They have gotten much better over the years and introduced a few different flavors. Like the protein powder, they use the same blend and have either deluxe bar for those looking for extra calories and they also make the lite bars for those looking to try and lose weight. The lite bars have half the calories and fat of the deluxe bars and are considered to be a great meal replacement. Whatever your goal is just make sure you don't rely solely on these nutritional protein bars.

Meso-Tech Bars by MuscleTech (Cookies & Cream, Peanut Butter Chocolate or Chocolate Chip Cookie) – great tasting bars packed with quality protein blends and a few amino acids for muscle building. Like any other bar do not consume more than 2 servings daily – remember these bars are mostly all high in sugar and saturated fat.

Muscle Milk Bars by CytoSport (chocolate Peanut Caramel) – these bars are fairly new on the market and don't really know how they are rated. I mentioned before that their protein powder and RTD's are phenomenal. I tasted these bars a few times and they were quite delicious. I like their ingredients and their protein blends. So in my opinion it's a good nutritional and tasting bar. Go ahead and grab one while your reading the rest of this book.

PowerBar Performance Bars by PowerBar Inc. – these bars are considered to be classified as energy bars rather than protein bars. Invented by an Olympic marathoner PowerBar was designed with endurance athletes in mind. These bars contain large amounts of carbohydrates to deliver a big boost of energy when needed. These bars also deliver many essential vitamins and minerals, along with some protein to help aid muscle growth, recovery and repair. However, like so many other bars, it contains quite a bit of sugar so make sure that you're active enough to burn it off.

Clif Bar by Clif Bar Inc. – another type of energy bar and a great product for all wakes of people. Clif Bars are made with all natural ingredients such as organic soy flour and soy protein. You can find these bars in almost every supermarket, deli, convenience store and other little mom and pop shops. Like the PowerBar, Clif Bars are designed to give you that boost of energy needed for a workout, race or any endurance type activity. It contains many nutrients, vitamins and amino acids and happens to taste pretty damn good. I enjoy the chocolate chip flavor but they make enough flavors for you to decipher which one you enjoy.

Balance Bars by the Balance Bar Food Company – another energy bar and quite popular. The Balance Bar approach is based on the 40-30-30 belief. That is 40% Carbohydrates, 30% Protein, and 30% Fat. It's the ideal bar for athletes who need that burst of energy. Since the bar contains little amounts of calories and carbohydrates it can be burned off fairly easy. The chocolate crisp flavor is delicious and low in sugar (12 grams), low in fat (6 grams) and has a fair amount of protein (15 grams).

These 10 protein and energy bars I have listed are once again just a few of the millions of products out there. I hope you enjoy at least one of the companies from the list above and if you don't I am more than positive that you will end up finding your ideal bar. Like protein powders and shakes, these bars should not be a substitute for a meal unless you have no other choice. They are high in sugar, calories, sodium, fat and carbohydrates so I recommend you control your intake to one or two bars at most per day. They can make a great snack for post and pre workouts since they give you the energy needed to sustain. Although numerous amounts of research debunk the idea that protein bars, protein shakes and protein diets build muscle, the theory and fascination is alive and is spoken of in most gyms, fitness centers and fitness facilities.

Part III – The Creatine & Glutamine Craze

Another one of those topics that people ask me about is what creatine is and which one do I recommend or use? Creatine Monohydrate is a nitrogen-containing substance that's produced naturally in your body and is found in such foods as meat (steak), chicken and fish. It is the building block for several amino acids, which themselves are the building blocks for protein synthesis. Over the past few years Creatine has been regarded as a necessity by all bodybuilders and even some athletes. Creatine is an expensive supplement and can have both negative and positive effects on the body. In essence Creatine stimulates muscle growth by increasing your energy levels – additional energy results in allowing your body to perform more work and in the process you can begin to lift heavier and gain some weight, size and muscle mass. Since creatine gets stored in the muscle it will begin to hold or retain more water in its cells and becomes "volumized" or what I call super-pumped. Your body is now holding more water and gives you a fuller and hydrated appearance. A negative effect of creatine is that since it retains much of the water in your body it is extremely important that you keep yourself constantly hydrated. I experienced an episode of dehydration during my creatine cycle and I don't want any of you to experience it at first hand. Your body shuts down and you are lucky if you have an ounce of energy to take another step. In addition make sure that your potassium intake is high so this way you don't cramp or get muscle spasms while engaging in physical activity. There is no preferred creatine supplement, and just like protein bars and powders every single manufacturer has an item on the shelf. When I was 20 I didn't have many choices like people have today. It was either powder form or syrup that gets dissolved once it hits your tongue. Now-A-days creatine comes in a variety of flavors, syrups, serums and even pill form (capsules) for easier digestion. Creatine has truly become one of the most popular supplements and an expensive one as well. Since all these products are not FDA approved then the only true evidence we have is ourselves. We have become the critics, supporters and promoters for almost all bodybuilding supplements. The reality of creatine is that it actually works and has some value. From my experience and from several human studies creatine can help weight lifters, bodybuilders and endurance athletes build muscle and gain strength. Creatine seems to give these athletes and professional bodybuilders an anaerobic energy boost, which enables them to lift more, run quicker while gaining strength and size. A word of advice – make sure that you cycle off creatine after a few weeks or a few months. You should never take creatine on a continuous basis for one full year. It will not get you any bigger and stronger; it will on the other hand give you kidney and liver problems and even lead to many episodes of dehydration, anxiety and stomach cramps (diarrhea). On top of all that it will also cost you a fortune to continue your use of creatine so be smart and cycle on and off so that way your body doesn't rely solely on the supplement and realizes that it has to continue producing the needed amount in your body on its own. The truth of the matter is that there is no real answer as to which creatine supplement works the best. Everybody is different and responds differently to creatine and other supplements. Like I constantly say, what works for one individual will not always work for you. I have seen many cases where it did more damage than help for so many and on the other hand it drastically changed people's physiques, strength and endurance levels so who knows how each person will respond to this supplement. Now that we have a basic knowledge and understanding of what creatine is and what it can do, let's discuss a few brands that I have used over the years and which I think are good.

Cell-Tech Hardcore by MuscleTech – this was my first creatine powder every used. It was and still is a great seller and an excellent product with lots of bodybuilders endorsing this product and company. I felt myself getting stronger almost instantly and even had a burst of energy that got me through those hard workouts. It comes in four flavors (Fruit Punch, Orange, Lemon-Lime and Grape) and they all taste good. I mixed two scoops daily with 16-20 oz of water and drank one upon waking up and the other either before or after my workout. My 4.5 pound container lasted me approximately 8 weeks and I followed the loading and maintenance stage. This becomes a bit difficult for those first using this product – the loading stage is done for the first five days and it's not a comfortable feeling. You need to drink this sweet, acidic powder in the morning when you wake up and then either before or after a workout. This was not the highlight of my day because after gulping it down in the early hours of the morning I found myself nauseous, full, and dehydrated and was left with a burning sensation in the back of my throat – YUCK. After your loading stage is over, you begin to appreciate what this product can deliver. However, I must warn you now to make sure you are consuming at least one gallon of water throughout the day for maximum absorption and hydration.

Phosphagen by EAS – this has been around for a while and is an excellent source of creatine. It is not an expensive supplement and is highly recommended. I enjoyed the taste and its ability to really give me that extra burst of needed energy. Like most other creatine formulas this also requires a loading phase for the first five days. Make sure you consume enough liquids throughout your day and throughout your workout sessions.

CytoSport Fast Twitch Powder Punch - once again I really happen to like this company and the products they put out. I used this particular brand and flavor about a year ago and really enjoyed it. It was easy to drink and I don't recall there was a loading phase and it was only supposed to be taken on training days. This bottle lasted me longer than the others and was overall a decent product at a decent price.

BSN Cell-Mass in Arctic Berry Blast Flavor – an expensive form of creatine but absolutely worth it. These red shiny bottles really know how to come through with superb products. This creatine is designed to promote size, strength, hardness, performance and recovery. It contains absolutely no sugar and has a nice taste to it. I recommended this brand to my trainers and my friends and they all enjoyed it and increased their strength.

Gaspari Nutrition Size On (Arctic Lemon Ice) – a fairly new product on the market and a bit different than other creatine formulas. My gym partner and I tried this at the same time and noticed an increase in strength and size within the first 48 hours. We were blown away at how potent this product really was. Size On provided longer bursts of energy with an intense mind blogging pump for the duration of our workouts. They developed some real complex ingredients that I will not even bother to mention in this creatine. Unlike many other creatine formulas and cell volumizers, this product was easy on the stomach, had no abdominal discomfort, no feeling of nausea and no trips to the bathroom. Give this product a try, you might actually enjoy it.

Universal Nutrition Creatine Powder – a good source of creatine because it is manufactured in Germany. From previous articles and debates, Germany "supposedly" produces real pure and filtered creatine ensuring maximum results. I tried it for a while in between my off cycles and was not too impressed with this particular brand. However, I know many others that totally enjoyed it so I guess it's more of a taste and results preference.

Six Star Muscle Professional Strength Creatine – when one of my trainers brought this item for the gym I looked at him and told him that he had much to learn. The bottle was labeled with a price tag of $24.99 and looked a bit weird. Not weird like damaged or something but more in the sense of I had never heard of that company. It was extremely high in sugar and gave me stomach cramps almost immediately. The sweet taste of fruit punch burned my throat and I stopped using it after only a week's use. I don't recommend this creatine for one of two reasons – one it was way too cheap and the old saying is you pay for what you get. The second was the fact that he purchased it at some small little local drug store (I think Rite Aid). Supplements like this should only be sold in vitamin stores, local gyms and fitness stores. Not a likeable and recommendable product.

Almost all of the above mentioned companies produce creatine in the form of capsules, pills, serums and tablets. I have never tried these creatine pills and serums and don't know many others who have. I guess some people feel more comfortable swallowing pills then mixing some powder blend. I won't get into specifics with these pills but I know that some are cheaper than others. The powder blends are extremely expensive and can put a damper on your pocket while the pills sell for cheaper. I once saw my client purchase 120 capsules for $17.99. I guess the only way to find out which works better is to actually try both items. Manufacturers are constantly introducing all new blends, formulas, pills, capsules and tablets as a means to appeal to every single interested person. These products, all of which we have tried once or twice, have people going crazy over and obsessed with. They have become so dependent on these products that they believe their progress cannot be reached without it. As mentioned with all the fat burning pills in a previous chapter, all these products I have listed so far and reviewed are not approved by the FDA and are not intended to diagnose, cure, treat or prevent any disease. So all of these huge manufacturers' consumers act as science experiments until the day that the Food and Drug Administration begins to either approve or ban these "so called" helpful supplements.

Glutamine, my personal favorite supplement, is an amino acid that actually delivers results and helps your body in many ways. According to the Wikipedia (The Free Encyclopedia on the internet) it claims that L-Glutamine has a variety of biochemical functions and many uses. Glutamine has been studied extensively over the past 10-15 years and has been shown to be useful in the treatment of serious illnesses, injury, trauma, burns, cancer and its treatment related side-effects as well as in wound healing for postoperative patients; sounds like we found the magic ingredient – the ultimate cure for all our problems. However, we are not that lucky yet. L-glutamine is mostly marketed as a supplement used for muscle growth, muscle recovery and to aid in protein synthesis in weigh training, weight lifting, bodybuilding and other sports which require endurance. When I started working out twice a day my muscles began to really endure soreness and each workout was getting harder and harder. Even with proper supplementation, rest and vitamins I needed something that wouldn't get me as sore. This huge bodybuilder in the gym asked me one day if I take L-Glutamine and my reply was what the hell is that? He told me to go home and google it and get your hands on it as soon as possible and watch what happens. Well a month later a few things happened once I began to use glutamine: (1) I had quicker recovery time, felt less sore and actually gained some muscle growth (2) I became an unofficial advocate for glutamine and recommended it to everyone who lifts weights seriously. Too bad I wasn't able to sign a deal with some big glutamine manufacturer and (3) I noticed that I was running out of money quicker. L-Glutamine in any form (pills, capsules or powder) and company is quite expensive and doesn't last for too long. Replenishment was needed every month or so and I decided to write this book to pay for my glutamine obsession. Today, L-glutamine comes in all sorts of ways: powder, capsules and tablets and is even found in many protein powders as an additive. Of course you can get glutamine from certain foods that you eat such as meats, fish, poultry, beans and many dairy products. I listed my all time three favorite glutamine supplements to better aid you in your decision on which one to take.

MHP Glutamine SR (sustained-Release) 1000g – I have used this particular glutamine product for almost three years and really enjoy it. It's a tasteless powder that you can easily add it to any protein shake, juice drink or water. It is considered to be a popular brand of glutamine and is used widely by many fitness professionals. I give it a thumbs up, except for the price. It is expensive......

PROLAB Nutrition Glutamine Powder 1000g – another good choice for those that want real pure glutamine. It is a flavorless and easy mixing formula for easy digestion. This brand is always expensive but I think it's worth the money.

Twinlab Amino Fuel 2000 – 150 tablets – a fairly reasonable price for this product and I have used it numerous of times. It comes in a tablet form so make sure you have no problem swallowing since these tablets are pretty big. I learned how to swallow these pills almost instantly after almost choking. Twinlab has been around for years and puts out real good quality products at reasonable prices. If you don't like the flavorless powders then go ahead and take these tablets. Only drawback is that you need to take at least 4-6 tablets daily, so that means your stash will need to be replenished quickly.

Chapter 12
Nutrition Today and Healthy Tomorrow

So chapter 11 was filled with important information regarding all those supplements we desperately yearn for and can't live without. So suppose they don't help you burn fat, build muscle, supply you with bursts of energy, then what actually does? The most logical answer is eating sensible in moderation and exercising. If you exercise regularly and follow some basic nutritional guidelines you should begin to feel good, look good and see results sooner than you think......It's as simple as that. If you don't know by now let me tell you – approximately 65% (as of 2005-2006 – numbers could have changed) of the U.S. population is overweight or obese. Millions, maybe even billions, of dollars has been poured into the economy in hopes of educating and promoting Americans of healthy and fit lifestyles. It is a long road and will require more awareness, more education and the help of each and every one of us. There are so many obstacles to eating well in America: people's busy lifestyles, the availability of convenience and healthy foods, huge portions, lack of information regarding nutrition and weight loss and the denial of people thinking they have a weight problem. All these obstacles are mostly over-looked and ignored by so many. You must take an initiative and begin to make changes immediately. It is never too late to improve your health, your concerns and your overall appearance. Heart attacks, diabetes, high blood pressure and high cholesterol are all on the rise and we need to start making changes. Changing your dietary habits at any age (young or old) can significantly improve the way you feel and even decrease your risk of chronic diseases.

To lose weight you must eat more. How can this actually make sense? While most people believe that in order to lose weight they must starve themselves and consume a cracker and a glass of water a day. You must eat more in a course of a day in small portions to constantly keep your metabolism active and working. A few key components for healthy living and losing weight are:

(1) Eat less Fat – many of today's trendy diets talk about keeping your fat intake to about 30% or less of your calories from fat consumed. By cutting back on fat you will control your weight, lower your risk of chronic illnesses and even have more energy throughout the day. Basically, you need to learn how to read labels and monitor your portions and replace foods high in fat with nutritional low-fat options. It is important to note that one gram of fat contains 9 calories. When consuming a meal or snack please take into consideration the calorie versus the calories from fat ratio.

(2) Eat less saturated fat – saturated fat clogs up your arteries just as much as cholesterol does. Minimize the amounts of saturated fat you consume daily and begin to make smart substitutions.

(3) Control, or cut back, on your portions – Americans love to eat and the bigger the portions the better it is for us. The American consumers are apparently becoming more and more demanding on value for their money. This has become a full blown epidemic of obesity and overweight – just because the mound of food is on your plate does not mean that you should devour it along with the plate. You have to become a smarter eater and know when to draw the line and call it quits. It starts with little changes and by the time you know it those huge portions will look way too big and you will start to control your desire to finish it.

(4) Drink plenty of water – water is one of your body's most important nutrients and is used for so many functions: keeping your skin moist, transports oxygen to your tissues, lubricates your joints and keeps you feeling good. The recommended amount that we always hear to drink is at least 8-12 ounce glasses, not including all other beverages. You will begin to visit the bathroom often to urinate and if you're drinking the right amount you will notice it to be clear and plentiful. You will release many toxins, sodium and other chemicals every time you urinate.

(5) Eat several meals a day – I mentioned this before and can't stress the importance of eating 4 to 6 meals a day. These meals can be small in portions, but will help tremendously in keeping your energy levels stable and controlled. The majority of people I know still stick to the traditional three-meals-a-day approach – a hearty breakfast, a huge lunch and a real filling dinner right before you go to bed. Eating these three meals and waiting hours before the next meal will cause you to feel sluggish, groggy and have sudden changes in your blood sugar levels. Your metabolism this way will not be as active as it should and can lead to weight gain. In addition, since you are only consuming three meals chances are that they are not as nutritious as they really should be – you just want to eat and get full so that way you can last until your next meal. I use to follow this approach and always found myself tired, sluggish and no energy. It wasn't after one year of working out that I found out how important it is to eat several meals a day. I was able to gain some size and muscle mass while constantly having my energy levels stable.

(6) Increase or boost your fiber intake – Fiber in your diet can help decrease hunger and help with weight loss. High-fiber foods generally require more chewing time, thus giving your body time to register when you are no longer hungry. In other words, it will decrease your chances of overeating since you will be fuller for a greater amount of time. Fiber is often classified into two categories: Insoluble fiber (those that don't dissolve in water) and Soluble Fiber (those that do dissolve in water). Insoluble fiber is usually found in wheat flour, wheat products, whole-grain breads and cereals, bran, nuts and many vegetables. Soluble fiber is found in foods such as oats, legumes (beans), peas, apples, citrus fruits, carrots, barley and psyllium. A high fiber diet can

also be beneficial to you because it lowers blood cholesterol levels, aids in weight loss, lowers your risk and chances of digestive conditions and also controls blood sugar levels. If you are having a tough time getting your recommended amounts of fiber then maybe you should begin taking fiber pills or capsules.

(7) Dedicate time for rest – sleep is extremely important for your body's overall ability to concentrate, remember information, perform mental tasks and even reduce the stress levels in your body. Stress can be related to many things and one of them being neglecting enough sleep. Your body requires a good amount of sleep (usually 6-8 hours) a night to sustain for your lives up and coming challenges, tasks and performance factors.

(8) Eat more fruits and vegetables – as previously noted, fruits and vegetables are a great source of fiber and even contain many vital antioxidants, vitamins, minerals and nutrients. Almost every diet promotes the consumption of fruits and vegetables eaten throughout the day. Most people, who I came across, that were successful at maintaining weight loss tend to eat more of these products than the average person.

(9) Drink Green Tea – studies over the past few years have concluded that green tea can help with weight loss. Considered to be one of the worlds most powerful and healthy fat burners, green tea has become extremely popular and is used frequently in almost all diet programs. Besides its ability to help burn fat, green tea has been linked to many studies all of which promote healthy living. Do a search on Google regarding Green Tea and see what comes up. I am sure all the information will be helpful and maybe even motivate you to start drinking loads of green tea.

(10) Decrease your sodium (salt) and sugar intake. To spice things up and add flavor to your food, use lemon, pepper and other spices. For those who have a sweet tooth, use a sugar substitute such as equal, splenda, stevia or even brown sugar. Some sugars are not clearly indicated on the list of ingredients. Here is a list, to name but a few, of sugars that may be unidentifiable to the average shopper:

- Alcohol sugars ("ol" endings, ie; sorbitol, mannitol, etc.)

- Artificial flavors

- Aspartame/NutraSweet (causes cravings and made from alcohol sugar)

- Bark sugar (also called Zylose)

- Barley malt

- Barley syrup

- Beet sugar

- Black Strap Molasses

- Brown rice syrup

- Cane juice

- Cane sugar

- Caramel coloring

- Corn sweetener

- Corn syrup

- Dextrose

- Disaccharides

- Evaporated cane juice

- Extracts (any type of flavor)

- Fructose (fruit sugar)

- Glucose (blood sugar)

- Granulated sugar

- Honey (any type of form)

- Invert sugar

- Lactose (milk sugar)

- Malted barley

- Maltose (malt sugar)

- Maple sugar

- Maple Syrup

- Milled sugar

- Modified food starch

- Molasses

- Monoglycerides

- "Natural Sweeteners" or "Naturally Sweetened"

- Nectar

- Olestra (made from sucrose)

- Pectin

- Powdered sugar

- Raw sugar

- Ribose

- Rice sugar

- Rice sweeteners

- Rice syrup

- Sorbitol (also called Hexitol)

- Sorghum (found in beer)

- Splenda

- Stevia

- Sucrose (table sugar)

- Unrefined sugar

- Vanillan

- Whey

- White sugar

- Xanthum gum

- Xylitol

- Zylose

Proper nutrition and proper supplementation (vitamins) are key components to healthy living. It is just absolutely amazing how your body, your looks and the way you feel almost instantly changes once nutritional awareness is introduced. Everyone has heard the popular saying "You are what you eat" and what a true saying it is. Making nutritional adjustments is no easy task and the best advice I can give someone is to make changes gradually. Trying to make too many changes quickly can leave you feeling overwhelmed, frustrated and even a bit skeptical. Instead, you must ease into nutrition, supplementation and exercise. Like anything else in this world we must start off easy with the constant pursuit of dedication, determination and possibility. The goals you set have to be realistic and always changing. If your goal was to lose 10 pounds then your next goal is to lose 10 more. Evaluate your past accomplishments because I am almost sure you have probably been successful in tackling many other difficult tasks. Reminding yourself of past accomplishments and goals can give you the much needed confidence and desire to make necessary changes that will ultimately lead to weight loss.

Before starting any weight loss program/regiment/routine, I recommend a quick visit to your local doctor's office. A short visit with all the necessary blood work and health assessment can definitely put you on the right path. Below you will find a nutritional program I wrote for my two clients when they asked what they should eat for a healthy lifestyle. I devoted my time and even made an appearance into their office to see what they have hidden in their refrigerator and closets. To my demise I confiscated all of their carbonated beverages (soda's), chocolate pudding and chocolate chip cookies. Instead, I gave them a shopping list containing many nutritional products and cases of water, low-fat yogurt and some fiber-grain cereals. I am not a nutritionist and would like to get that straight. This program was written for them just to act as a guide and in no means should this be used to cure or diagnose obesity, overweight or any other illness. Rather, this is just a little of the knowledge I gained from meeting with numerous nutritionists, doctors and fitness professionals. Just to leave you off with a side note; these two clients of mine have been following my program and are noticing major changes. One of them being more active and less tired, while the other one is feeling great daily and having the coordination and concentration needed to get through long hard work days. They are working out constantly and have become more health conscious than I ever expected them to be. Good job guys and keep up the work...........

David & Ben

Here are some general rules regarding general nutrition that you guys must apply:

1) Maintain consistency – be consistent in your diet

2) Eat several meals a day – try to keep your energy levels constant

3) Eat balanced meals – Eat a balance of protein, slow-digesting carbohydrates, healthy fats and vegetables

4) Consume adequate protein – protein is the most reliable tool for muscle growth

5) In regards to slow-digesting carbohydrates – here are a few examples (sweet potatoes, oatmeal, brown rice, whole-grain breads and pastas, quinoa and fruits)

6) Eat healthy foods – use your better judgment

7) Avoid trans fats – hydrogenated oil or partially hardened vegetable oil

8) Eat plenty of fiber or take a fiber supplement – fiber is in some fruits and vegetables, legumes, nuts and seeds

9) Drink enough water

10) Learn to read labels

11) Take a multivitamin daily – taking this vitamin daily ensures that you get all the nutrients you need for optimal gains

In order to lose weight you have to increase your metabolism (you do this by eating a lot of meals in a day), exercise (both weight training and cardiovascular) and you have to make sure that all sugars, salt and carbohydrates are being consumed in moderation. Your meals should be eaten every two to three hours and they should be both nutritional and filling. Cut out all carbonated beverages, Snapple's, sugar juices, etc... Water should become your only form of liquid. If you eat in a controlled fashion and watch what you eat, weight loss should begin to occur. Here is a sample of a normal eating regiment....

Breakfast (Meal #1) – usually eaten between 7am-9am

Egg whites (omelet, scrambled, etc...) – 3 to 6 eggs

Whole Wheat Toast/Seven Grain bread with butter/jelly/low-fat cheese

Or

Oatmeal

Or

Cereal (any type of fiber/grain cereal)

Fresh fruits

Cottage Cheese or yogurt

*** You can have any type of beverage (tea, coffee – just try to use some sugar substitute)

Meal #2 – this is known as a snack – usually eaten right between breakfast and lunch

This is usually a light snack and is meant to increase your metabolism. It can consist of any of the following:

Yogurt

Smoothie or Protein Shake

Protein bar or any nutritional bar

Fruit – any type of fruits you desire

Almonds/nuts/cashews/etc...

Lunch (Meal #3) – This is usually eaten between the hours of 12pm-2pm

Grilled Chicken salad

Tuna salad/tuna wrap

Sushi (if you can try to get brown rice sushi)

Any type of salad with low fat dressing

Fish (salmon/tuna/snapper) – make sure it's grilled or broiled

*** You want to make sure you are eating a good lunch so that it can keep your energy levels high and constant throughout the whole day

Meal #4 - Snack – usually eaten after lunch and before dinner or a workout

Once again this is a small snack and it's just meant for you to keep your metabolism high and working. By doing this you will begin to burn more calories and hopefully lose weight. Your body will be busy working and burning fat and this is a good thing.

Meal #5 – Dinner – usually eaten between 6pm-8pm and is your last meal for the night

Whatever your wife makes for dinner is fine. Once again try to minimize or cut down all your sodium (salt) intake and unnecessary sugars. If you are having either rice or potatoes use the following:

A substitute for white rice – brown rice/buckwheat/organic rice

A substitute for potatoes – sweet potatoes – they are easier to digest and break down

*** Along with this eating regiment you must do following: (1) Exercise (Fitness By kobi, biking, walking, etc…) (2) Sleep well – this is important so that you let your body recover properly and function normally and (3) dedication – you are your biggest critic so commit yourself for a month and give it all you have. This is your life, your health and your challenge.

Chapter 13
Fitness Finale (Summary and Closing Thoughts)

"Fitness is not a luxury, it is a necessity" – I am hoping by now that you have gained a sense of knowledge, understanding and a yearning desire for what fitness has to offer. Aside from the good looks and big biceps, getting fit and healthy is at the forefront of our generation. We have seen many gains and accomplishments throughout so far and I believe that we can do much more. Olympic records are broken, competitive sports are viewed by many, body transformations are becoming common, and the overall pursuit of perfection is being challenged daily. I expect my readers to follow some basic principles as a means to achieve their goals. No matter what your goals are and what you strive for, remember that the toughest task will be challenging yourself. Each day brings us new challenges, some days we find success and others we may fall short but in the end we realize that attaining this success requires patience, dedication and an absolute passion. The game of fitness and healthy living does not require you to have a P.H.D. or even be a college graduate; it requires you to understand and learn basic information. To make progress and begin to actually see results, you've simply got to know what you're doing and where you're going. Evaluate your goals as you see fit and embark on this wonderful path of becoming healthy. A good friend of mine once told me something that I will never forget – "you don't need to sleep in order to dream." We all can strive for perfection if we really tried and what better way trying then fitness and health.

Knowledge Only Builds Inspiration

Keep On Believing In yourself

TESTIMONIALS

"Absolutely a great trainer and a powerful motivator. I enjoy all of your training sessions and look forward to the next one. Thank you for giving me the confidence I need to go on."

Florina Krupnitsky, M.S. – CCC – SLP (Speech Language Pathologist)

"You have that great combination of looks, knowledge, passion and commitment that really attracts people. Let's face it, your body is perfection and you clearly possess a great amount of understanding about what works. Good luck with all that you do and hopefully this book will teach so many others."

Brian T. Keliher (client of mine for three years)

"I am extremely happy with the last couple of months training with you. I feel better than I felt in years; my body feels like it's starting to make drastic changes, while my endurance levels are way up. I look forward to all our workouts and even more anxious for the upcoming book and secrets."

Morris Beyda (client of mine for 2 years and personal friend)

"Wow – your knowledge, experience and advice on weight training are a great tool for almost anyone interested in fitness. You have a real sense of knowledge and passion about fitness and nutrition. Good luck with all that you do. I don't doubt your success for a minute and can't wait to get my own copy of the book."

Scott Losche (Personal Trainer, Division I baseball coach and my old time favorite training partner)

"I feel great. I feel a huge difference in my body already and extremely excited to come and see more results. Thanks Kobi, I couldn't have done it without your help and inspiration."

Lillian Gadeh-Betesh (female client of mine for a year and my number 1 PR girl)

"Thank you so very much….it means a lot to me knowing that you are helping me achieve my goal towards optimum health and a body to kill for (lol). I hope we can get to that level together. You are my inspiration and a great friend and trainer."

Shelley Kabilu (client of mine for three months and together we are making a complete body transformation)

"Thanks for your help and advice Kobi. You really seem genuinely interested and passionate about what you are doing and it's absolutely amazing to see that. I know this book will be a great seller and I better get a signed copy (lol)."

Michael Lookwood (client of mine for 2 months and extremely dedicated since he met me)

"Just an overall superb trainer and a great person to be around. You seem to always know the answers and I have learned so much from you over the past year and a half."

Allen Razam (Certified Fitness Trainer and one of my trainers at my studio)

"Kobi's knowledge when it comes to fitness is out of this world! He addresses the body as a machine but also as a work of art. The results, a defined and beautifully symmetrical creation! I really respect his vision and enjoy the workouts"

Ashley Bryce Sharaby (client of mine for 2 years now and a well-respected registered nurse in NYC)

"When is there a time that you don't know something regarding fitness? You are like a fitness god (lol) and I respect your work ethics." Thanks for always giving me accurate and knowledgeable advice."

Isaac Z. (client of mine for a year and a great mentor, friend and father figure)

"You seem like you can be the voice to begin making positive changes in the realm of fitness. You have a true sense of pride, commitment, determination and love for fitness and health. Good luck in all that you pursue."

Reuven Noiman (a true friend, financial partner and my brother)

"You're a remarkable trainer and even a greater motivational speaker. You seem to always know what to say to make me still come and train."

Joe Bosco (training partner of mine while I was competing and a great role model)

These are just a few of the thousands of testimonials and quotes I receive monthly. I love to always hear positive, as well as negative, input, ideas and criticisms. Not everyone is always going to listen to what you say or do and at times they will even question you. Thus, I make sure to always listen to my clients and never place myself above them. We are all equal and all want the same things, so why not work as a team and achieve our goals more rapidly. Till this day I still find myself learning more and more about the amazing world of fitness and healthy living. I accept criticism as a form of education and work to strengthen my weaknesses, my flaws and my overall perception and views on certain topics.

Since the grand opening of my fitness facility in 2007, clients, friends and my staff suggested that we place a huge board with before and after photos. It has now been a year and I still have not put up a board nor have pictures of my clients. Most people I know, including many of these readers, love to see before and after photos along with some captions and bits of information. We feel like by maybe seeing others achieve goals and success then maybe we can too. I, on the other hand, do not believe that these photos are necessary. Who better than yourself to know how you look now and how you looked before? You are your biggest critic, fan and nemesis. The battles you endured and still enduring are not just memories and recollections, rather they are real-life. I don't need fancy photos and a huge board to display my talent. Fitness is my passion and my absolute love and with every client that I change, inspire, educate and interact with is better than any before and after photos. I admire my hard work and the hard work of my clients and I reward them, rather they reward themselves, with the passage to being healthier, fit and happier. In addition, all those before and after photos we see and enjoy reading how much weight someone lost are not always true. Remember, fitness is a great profession but can also be a great money maker so gym owners and trainers will do almost anything to promote themselves. Before and after photos have worked wonders for so many but for me I still always strive and aspire for perfection in each and every one of my clients. I don't need photos. My clients make up the collage on my wall, in my heart, in my mind and in my presence.

About the Author

Kobi Noiman began weight training at the late age of 19 years old. Almost in decent shape and active in sports, it wasn't until his first year of college that he began to embark on a lucrative and gratifying profession: Fitness Trainer. A dedicated weight lifter and bodybuilder fanatic, Kobi made sure to always hit the gym, educate himself on the sport as well as challenge himself almost daily. He really took the saying "no pain no gain" to its ultimate level and never once gave up nor complained.

Today Kobi is a well-respected and well-known fitness trainer. His expertise and dedication regarding fitness are second to none. He has evolved as an elite trainer who has one goal in mind: changing the lives of others. His success comes from his love of fitness and his overall manifestations of each and every client he touches. Since the opening of his fitness studio in Brooklyn, New York (Fitness by Kobi) in 2007, it has become an elite fitness studio with great trainers, consultants and nutritionists who pride themselves on being leaders in the fitness industry. Kobi is certified by the American College of Sports Medicine, the International Sports Sciences Association (ISSA) and the American Council on Exercise (ACE). He has been featured in numerous fitness magazines (exercise for Men) and written a great amount of articles and excerpts for several publications and bodybuilding magazines. His knowledge on fitness is a staple in the industry and with the hopes of making this book a great seller he has one vision: to revolutionize the fitness industry by making millions more aware, more educated, more dedicated and more motivated. This is only a glimpse of what is going to come. I will educate everyone and begin to make some serious advancements in the near future regarding fitness and healthy living. Hang on, be strong, stay confident, stay competitive and always maintain that passion and desire.

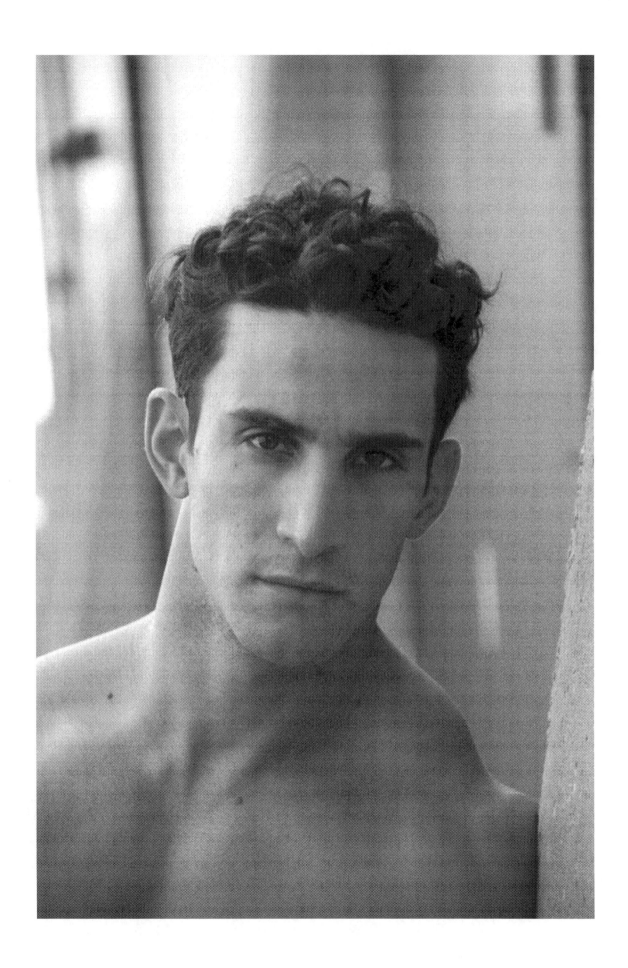

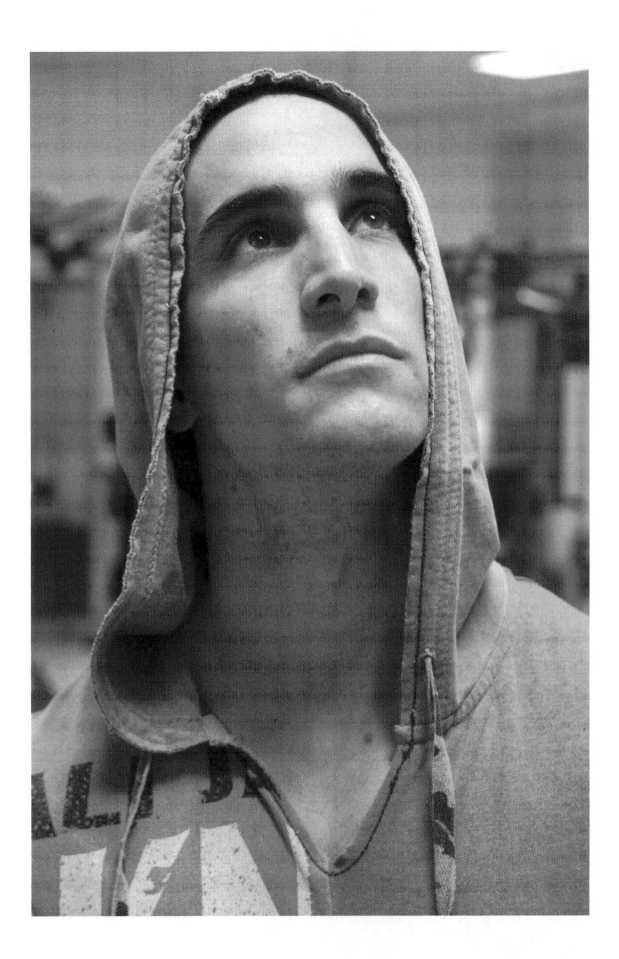

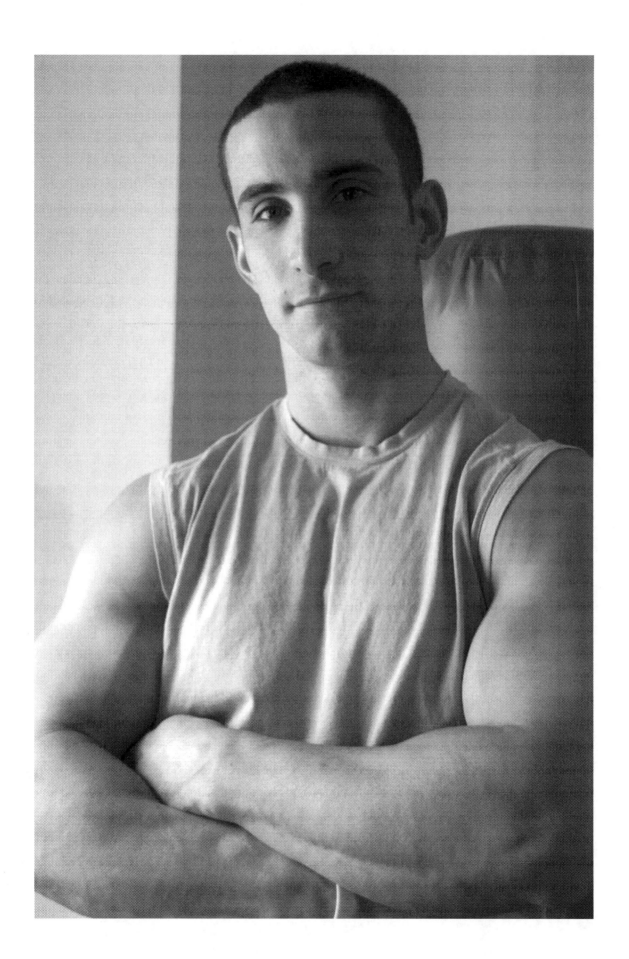

Credits

I would like to thank all of my friends, family, trainers and clients for making this book possible. I could have never done it without your support, encouragement and understanding. This book is especially dedicated for my mother, the single most important woman in my life, who went through more than anyone can imagine. I thank you for every second that I breathe. In addition, I would also like to thank two other people: my brother Reuven and my girlfriend Ashley. My brother has been by my side from the beginning and became my number one Chief Financial Advisor. My girlfriend Ashley, wow where can I start. You spent numerous amounts of hours reading and editing this book to make sure it was perfect. You truly are a remarkable young lady with strong characteristics. I guess that's what you get when you date a bodybuilder. Thank you all once again and I will continue to promote my efforts in revolutionizing the entire fitness industry.

Additional Credits

"FITNESS IS NOT A LUXURY, IT IS A NECESSITY" ™

www.fitnessbykobi.com

(Please feel free to view my website for all upcoming events, workout
routines, photo gallery, blog and products for sale)

Once Again I will like to thank all of my family, friends, clients and supporters for sticking by
my side and helping me pursue the making of this book. I value each and every one of you
and will continue to promote my services and my knowledge with all those who need help.
Fitness and healthy living should never be underestimated or under appreciated. A special
thanks to the following people:

Jana Sanford – my photographer, my client and a great person to be around. If you have any
questions or need to book her, please do not hesitate to contact her at janasanford@gmail.
com or check out her website: http://www.janasanford.com/

Bobby Filipov – Certified Personal Trainer and a highly known and respected athlete. Born in
Bulgaria, Bobby was a Track & Field champion and a celebrity in his country. He is extremely
talented, perfectly conditioned and absolutely takes pride in the way he trains. The chapters
regarding legs and Abdominals were done by Bobby, and I would like to thank him for doing
it all on short notice. He is a great trainer, father, husband and an overall unique person.
Bobby, I sincerely thank you and wish you all the luck in the world. If you need to contact
Bobby for any fitness related issue please do not hesitate to reach out to him: His email is
bobbyfitness@hotmail.com.

Allen Razam – one of my first original trainers at my studio. Allen saw it all – the up's, the
down's and the excitement. A special thanks to you Allen for sticking by my side and helping
turn my place into a studio of elite personal trainers. Originally from Israel, (my home town
as well) Allen was a renowned wrestling champion, swimming champion and a fitness model.
He has a great amount of knowledge regarding fitness and he continues to shine and work
his ranks up in the fitness industry.

Eyal Bruchim – if you are reading this part Eyal just wanted to let you know I always talk about
you and never forget you. Eyal is a special friend to me and worked at my studio as a personal
trainer. An ex-Israeli soldier and trainer to the Israeli Navy Seals, Eyal worked for me for
about a year and developed some really good relations with the staff and the clients. Almost
instantly his impact was felt by many of his clients and he is also responsible for helping many

of them reach their goals and drastically change their lives. I learned my share of things from you and extremely proud to call you my friend. Good luck Eyal......

Reuven Noiman – my financial partner, my friend, my brother and my role model. You are a unique and inspirational person to be around. I would have never gotten this far if it wasn't for you seeing potential in me. You have a great gift and even a better sense of people's capacities, potentials and limitations. You supported me and pushed me when no one else did. I truly owe you all the success and fame that I have achieved this far. You will always continue to shine and bring out the best in me. Reuven, I love you and want every reader to know that having a brother like you by their side is like having the world at the palms of your hands. Thanks brother.......

Ashley Sharaby – wow, where do I begin. You made this book possible by staying up all those nights helping me edit, write, read, and so much more. You stuck by my side and always encouraged me to never give up and to follow my dream. Well it's now official and one book is under our belts. What's next? I know – another book (LOL). You are my true soul mate, my girlfriend, my reason to live and most of all, my friend. I love you baby and dedicate this book to you and to let you know that this is just the beginning to the rest of our lives together.

Riki Noiman-Marzano – for those who don't know this happens to be my mother. Mom, I thank you every day that I breathe for bringing me into this life and providing for both your children. You are an incredible lady with a heart of gold. You are so much concerned at times with the overall activities in your children's lives that you over look your own pleasure. You stuck by my side and allowed me to shine and evolve and in return I want to thank you and tell you that I love you with every beat of my heart. I cannot think of anything wrong that you have done in your life to better aid your children and your career. Your friends, family and all others who you touched and inspired have nothing but the kindest and sincere words to describe you. They are beautiful people and will always continue to speak highly of you. Mom, please accept this book as a thank you for all the good you have done to all.

Jerry Marzano – my father who passed away from complications of cancer on July 31st, 2007. May you rest in peace and enjoy the heavens above. You were a great man and a caring father and husband. I appreciate all that you have done for me and how you made me understand the important things in life. These things you always related to were non-materialistic. Rather, they were the necessities to all human form – water, air and health. I loved listening to you while you spoke in a firm tone teaching me with such great passion and vision. You always made me see things differently and I wish I had one last chance to say goodbye and thank you for all that you have done. You died on a Tuesday at 10 PM and I saw you close your eyes for the last time. I know you are in a better place and it will be selfish of me to ask for you back but I want you to know that if it wasn't for you in my life I have no idea as to where I would now be. You provided for me, fought for me and always pointed me in the right direction. Seeing me get hurt was something you cannot deal with and so you made sure that I never did. I love you more than words can say and I am happy to know that I saw you one last time before you passed and was even able to thank to you and share a few words. When I carried you up the stairs to my gym after your Chemo treatment and seeing you smile while we sat and spoke about random things was the last good memory of you in my mind. I had my share of turbulence and downfalls but I want you to know that I never gave up and always thought of you where ever I was. Jerry, I love you and hope that one day we can meet and share more fond memories, stories and success. I love you Dad and will remember you always and forever.

In addition to all the people I have listed, I want to thank each and every person that I have inspired through this book. My clients, friends and supporters I thank you guys as well. This is only the beginning of what's more to come and how I will try my absolute hardest to revolutionize the fitness industry and make millions aware of healthy lifestyle and healthy living. Thank you and good luck to all.

KEEP ON BELIEVING IN YOURSELF